Children Exposed to Violence

Children's exposure to violence (CEV) in their home, their community, and our society has finally been recognized as a serious mental health, social, and public health problem. This book highlights a summary of relevant current research, practice, and policy issues. It is the third in a series to help provide current state-of-the-science information to stimulate awareness, research, and best practices in the field.

This book provides chapters concerning the physiological effects of violence on children, its effects on behavioral and emotional functioning, and differences between boys and girls. Current interventions for children and families, such as innovative programs that are both home based as well as community based, are described. Promising and evidence-based practices are presented to provide the most recent approaches to helping children recover from the trauma of the abuse.

The chapters in this book provide greater awareness of the issues involved with CEV, stimulate additional research, improve practice techniques, lead to more evidence-based programs for both intervention as well as prevention, and help initiate a national priority to eliminate violence in the home and community.

This book was published as a special issue of the *Journal of Emotional Abuse*.

Robert Geffner is Founding President of the Family Violence and Sexual Assault Institute and Founding President of Alliant International University's (AIU) Institute on Violence, Abuse, and Trauma (IVAT). He is also currently Clinical Research Professor of Psychology at the California School of Professional Psychology, AIU, San Diego, CA.

Dawn Alley Griffin holds a joint appointment with Alliant International University's Center for Forensic Studies as a Research Associate and with the Center for Undergraduate Education as a faculty member and the coordinator of the criminal justice and the psychology programs.

James Lewis III is a clinical neuropsychologist and nationally certified school psychologist. Currently, he teaches program development to systems of acute response to children exposed to violence, and the effects of trauma on a child's developmental processes. He serves as a program consultant to New Opportunities Inc.

Children Exposed To Violence

Current Issues, Interventions and Research

Edited by Robert Geffner, Dawn Griffin
and James Lewis III

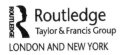 Routledge
Taylor & Francis Group
LONDON AND NEW YORK

First published 2009 by Routledge
2 Park Square, Milton Park, Abingdon, Oxon, OX14 4RN

Simultaneously published in the USA and Canada
by Routledge
270 Madison Ave, New York NY 10016

Routledge is an imprint of the Taylor & Francis Group, an informa business

Transferred to Digital Printing 2010

© 2009 Edited by Robert Geffner, Dawn Griffin and James Lewis III

Typeset in Times by Value Chain, India.

British Library Cataloguing in Publication Data
A catalogue record for this book is available from the British Library

ISBN10: 0-7890-3827-7 (h/b)
ISBN10: 0-7890-3828-5 (p/b)
ISBN13: 978-0-7890-3827-2 (h/b)
ISBN13: 978-0-7890-3828-9 (p/b)

CONTENTS

CURRENT INTERVENTION

Notes on Contributors

Su Shen Atta has over twenty years of experience in the field of domestic violence. She has served as the Program Supervisor of PACT Family Peace Center's Haupoa Family Component for the last twelve years.

Kimberly D. Becker is a clinical psychology postdoctoral fellow at the Johns Hopkins School of Medicine. Her research and clinical interests include child and adolescent psychopathology, evidence-based treatments, and family violence.

Dolores Subia BigFoot is an enrolled member of the Caddo Nation of Oklahoma and is an Assistant Professor in the Department of Pediatrics, University of Oklahoma Health Sciences Center. Dr. BigFoot directs the Indian Country Child Trauma Center.

Steven F. Bucky is Professor of Psychology, the Director of Professional Training, and the Interim Systemwide Dean at the California School of Professional Psychology, Alliant International University, San Diego, CA.

Caroline Cashman is a graduate student at the California School of Professional Psychology at Alliant International University, San Francisco, CA.

Linda Chamberlain is the Founder Director of the Alaska Family Violence Prevention Project with the State of Alaska Department of Health and Social Services. She earned her doctoral degree from Johns Hopkins University and a Masters of Public Health from the Yale University School of Medicine. She holds affiliate faculty positions with Johns Hopkins University and the University of Alaska.

David Chavis is President of the Association for the Study and Development of Community. He is internationally recognized for his work in the implementation, support, and evaluation of community initiatives including a distinguished career award from the American Psychological Association.

Elena P. Cohen is the director of the Safe Start Center at JBS International. The Center coordinates training and technical assistance, develops resources and publications, and convenes national and regional meetings to support the Safe Start Initiative. She previously directed the National Child Welfare Resource Center for Family-Centered Practice to provide technical assistance and consultation as well as develop and disseminate resources to State and Tribal child welfare agencies.

Abigail Gewirtz is Assistant Professor in the Department of Family Social Science and the Institute of Child Development at the University of Minnesota. Her research focuses on parenting and adjustment among traumatized children and on the development and implementation of evidence-based interventions for child trauma.

Hilary Hahn is an Associate Research Scientist at the National Center for Children Exposed to Violence at the Yale Child Study Center. Ms. Hahn coordinates national evaluation of the Child Development Community Policing (CD-CP) program and currently provides programmatic and evaluation consultation to developing and continuing CD-CP sites.

Nicolette Howells is currently a doctoral candidate in clinical psychology at Northern Illinois University.

Attorney Serena Noel Hulbert received Bachelor of Arts Degrees in Sociology/Criminal Justice and Philosophy from Valparaiso University, a Juris Doctorate from the John Marshall Law School, and possesses an active Wisconsin law license. She provides national training and technical assistance on a variety of issues confronting professionals working with children and families exposed to violence. Since 2002, she has worked with jurisdictions and national partners under the Office of Juvenile Justice and Delinquency Prevention's National Safe Start Project Grant, U.S. Department of Justice. Attorney Hulbert currently provides assistance to a variety of jurisdictions around the country, consulting on child welfare and family violence system process improvements through Hulbert Consulting Firm. Through her law practice, Hulbert Law Offices, LLC, she represents children and families in a variety of legal matters and is currently developing a pilot project with Dr. Karen Hulbert of the Medical College of Wisconsin and Jim Maro, President/CEO of the St. Rose Youth and Family Center of Milwaukee, WI, to assess and improve, among other things, the provision of comprehensive mental and physical health care and legal services to abused and neglected adolescents in out-of-home care.

Mary M. Hyde is a Senior Managing Associate with the Association for the Study and Development of Community. She is a community psychologist with 15 years of research and practice experience in various public interest issues.

Kata Issari has been working in the field of sexual and domestic violence for 25 years. She holds a Masters in Social Work currently serves as the Program Director of the Family Peace Center, a domestic violence intervention program of Parents and Children Together.

Kristen Kracke is the Safe Start Initiative Coordinator and program manager for the U.S. Department of Justice's Office of Juvenile Justice and Delinquency Prevention (OJJDP). Ms. Kracke developed and manages the national Safe Start initiative for the prevention, systems response, and treatment of children exposed to violence. Her areas of expertise include the development of collaborative systems change efforts to improve policy and practice for children and families, especially for those children and families exposed to violence.

Yvette H. Lamb is a former Senior Managing Associate with the Association for the Study and Development of Community.

Alan Lincoln is a Professor of Clinical Psychology in the California School of Professional Psychology of Alliant International University. He is also the Director of the Center for Autism Research, Evaluation, and Service in San Diego, California.

Gloria Mathis is a fifth-year graduate student in clinical psychology at the University of Hawaii-Manoa. Her research and clinical interests are in the area of children's mental health with a focus on the effects of family violence.

Amanuel Medhanie is a graduate student in the Department of Educational Psychology at the University of Minnesota, in the Quantitative Methods in Education track, focusing on statistics. He is currently a graduate research assistant in a research project focusing on high school mathematics curricula and college mathematics performance.

Charles W. Mueller is a Full Professor in social and clinical psychology in the Department of Psychology, University of Hawaii at Manoa. His research and applied work, focused on health, children's mental health, and aggression and violence, incorporates ideas and approaches from both areas of psychology.

Alan Rosenbaum is full professor in clinical psychology at Northern Illinois University and the Center for the Study of Family Violence and Sexual Assault.

Kristin W. Samuelson is an Assistant Professor at the California School of Professional Psychology at Alliant International University, San Francisco, CA.

Samuel Y. Song is an Assistant Professor of School Psychology at the University of North Carolina-Chapel Hill. His research program is called the Protective Peer Ecology Research Project. It consists of developing a model of effective bullying prevention and intervention in low-resource schools, and the development and evaluation of an innovative school bullying program.

Karen Callan Stoiber is Professor and Director of the School Psychology Program at the University of Wisconsin-Milwaukee. She has research interests in the area of evidence-based prevention and intervention, early literacy, problem-solving collaborative consultation, function-based assessment, and systems reform. She works collaboratively with state education, mental health, head start agencies, and school districts to promote evidence-based practices.

Steve Stride is an Assistant Professor in the Graduate Psychology Program and the Director of the Counseling Center at Trevecca Nazarene University. He has a diplomate in clinical psychology with an emphasis in marriage and family therapy as well as in history.

Staci Suzuki has worked as a group facilitator with both children and adults throughout her career. Her work has included domestic violence intervention, program management, special education services, and the delivery of cognitive-behavioral therapy. She is currently a treatment coordinator and licensed psychologist at Alvarado Parkway Institute in San Diego, CA.

Sadie Willmon-Haque is an enrolled member of the Western Delaware Nation of Oklahoma and is a doctoral candidate in the University of Oklahoma Counseling Psychology program.

Acknowledgments

We would like to acknowledge the efforts in the editing of the Think Tank report provided by Hillary Hahn at the Yale Child Study Center. In addition, Elena Cohen was instrumental in helping to organize the Think Tank as well as providing feedback on the report. Their comments and summaries were used in the Think Tank report, which was incorporated into the Introduction to this book. In addition, the participants of the CEV Think Tank provided insightful feedback and discussion regarding the issues presented in the Introduction. Their continued work and important contributions to the field have helped to create more awareness ness, research, promising practices, and policy recommendations. It should also be noted that the Think Tank and this book would not have been produced without the efforts and dedication of the National Center for Children Exposed to Violence, and Kristen Kracke of the Office of Juvenile Justice and Delinquency Prevention. Ms. Kracke's contributions to the field and to the work presented in this book have been invaluable. A special thank you is also given to Kristie Zoller for combining the Think Tank notes. A few other Alliant International University doctorate students transcribed and helped to compile the notes from the Think Tank, including Jessica Romo. We appreciate their efforts and time.

INTRODUCTION

Children Exposed to Violence: An Often Neglected Social, Mental Health, and Public Health Problem

Robert Geffner
Dawn Alley Griffin
James Lewis, III

Children's exposure to violence (CEV) in their home, their community, and our society has finally been recognized as a serious mental heath, social, and public health problem. Increased research, publications, funding, and focus on this issue have occurred in the past 8–10 years, and CEV has been given increased attention in a few identified communities; however, it has yet to be designated as a national priority. To help move the field forward, Alliant International University's Institute on Violence, Abuse, and Trauma hosted a Think Tank on "Children Exposed to Violence" in the Fall of 2006 at the 11th International Conference on Violence, Abuse, and Trauma in San Diego, California. This Think Tank was sponsored by the Office of Juvenile Justice and Delinquency Prevention (OJJDP) and the National Center for Children Exposed to Violence (NCCEV). A group of 28 recognized subject matter experts from research, practice, policy, academia, government, and nonprofit organizations participated in this effort to bring a cadre of professionals together for face-to-face discussions on the status of CEV as a critical component of a national strategy to protect children from the risks associated with traumatic exposure to violence. The primary focus of the Think Tank concerned the necessary strategy directions required for positive and lasting system changes in policy, research, education, training, and intervention. This special volume highlights a summary of relevant current research, practice, and policy issues as discussed during the Think Tank, presented at the 11th International Conference, or completed subsequent to the conference. The present chapter summarizes the main goals of the

Think Tank, the gaps in the topic areas of CEV, and the recommendations outlined at the Think Tank. It also introduces the chapters in this book and their relation to the different aspects of the Think Tank conclusions. This volume is the third in a series to help provide current state-of-the-science information to stimulate awareness, research, and best practices in the field (see Geffner, Igelman, & Zellner, 2003; Geffner, Jaffe, & Sudermann, 2000).

THINK TANK GOALS AND FRAMEWORK

One major outcome of the Think Tank was to identify the key issues needed to help advance the field of CEV. Those identified were: (a) defining and promoting strategies that expand the direction of system responsiveness to families experiencing violence; (b) identifying academic, research, and practice alliances to support evidence-based and promising practices service development and implementation; (c) agreeing on how to best coordinate efforts and develop an infrastructure for building an effective continuum of care for children exposed to violence and their families; and (d) determining information needs and how best to disseminate state-of-the-science and applied knowledge about CEV.

Three central principles provided a framework for the discussions at the Think Tank. First, it is important to take a public health perspective wherein the public health implications and consequences of adverse childhood experience are recognized and understood (e.g., the effects of intimate partner violence (IPV) on the adult victims and the children exposed have been linked to numerous adverse physical health issues, including back pain, peptic ulcers, asthma, diabetes, cardiovascular problems, and HIV/AIDS) (Anda et al., 2006; Felitti et al., 1998; Groves, Augustyn, Lee, & Sawires, 2002). Stride, Geffner, and Lincoln (in this book) provide research on the physiological effects of trauma and stress reactions in adults related to CEV. The traumatic mental health, behavioral, and social effects for CEV are addressed in this book by several researchers (e.g., Gewirtz & Medhanie; Samuelson & Cashman). Second, utilizing an ecological framework, Song and Stoiber (this book) and Suzuki, Geffner, and Bucky (this book), consider the individual, family, community, and societal factors in designing research, intervention, and prevention programs The third principle focused on adopting a child-centered approach to the family dynamics as essential to understanding CEV. Good examples of this type of application are the Safe from the Start initiative described in the chapters in this book (see Hyde,

Lamb, & Chavis; Kracke & Cohen) as well as in some other community-based programs (see Becker, Mathis, Mueller, Issari, & Atta; Chamberlain).

Current research, as reflected by the chapters in this volume, identifies a theoretical shift from single- to multi-factor interrelated causes that has occurred in the field of IPV and CEV (see Howells & Rosenbaum, this book; Kracke & Hahn, this book; Stith, Smith, Penn, Ward, & Tritt, 2004). Promising programs have been created to prevent IPV; however, research to evaluate the effectiveness of these programs has not progressed significantly, often due to the lack of collaborative relationships among practitioners, researchers, and policymakers, as well as their philosophical differences (Geffner & Rosenbaum, 2002; Stith et al., 2004). In the present volume, recent research that has focused on evaluating the outcome and effectiveness of intervention or prevention programs are presented as potential models that can be utilized by others (e.g., this book see Becker et al.; Chamberlain; Hyde et al.; Song & Stoiber). The chapters by Chamberlain, Hulbert, and Song and Stoiber highlight the utilization of outcome data to help design or modify intervention and prevention programs to link the findings of researchers, advocates, and practitioners. Becker et al. and Willmon-Haque and Bigfoot (this book) address the importance of including strategies that attempt to ensure that cultural factors are not only considered but also incorporated into the research and programs related to CEV.

Ideological issues and differences among the various constituencies have been a factor hindering the understanding of CEV and the empirical advancement of the field (e.g., Geffner & Rosenbaum, 2002). It is important that we directly address professional and discipline variations in nomenclature, style, and practice, while attempting to bridge ideological and philosophical differences. Therefore, the Think Tank invited a cadre of subject matter experts from divergent disciplines to come together and contribute their perspectives on four topic areas within the field of CEV: practice, policy, training, and research/evaluation. The following section provides an introduction with respect to key issues discussed during the Think Tank. Definitions, measurement, incidence, and prevalence were issues raised at the beginning of the discussions, and these were followed by a discussion of the service gaps and attention to underserved needs.

DEFINITIONS

Definitions of maltreatment, violence, and exposure to violence vary depending upon the system that is discussing or dealing with the issue.

Healthcare professionals, attorneys, researchers, and practitioners often use the definition most associated with their field. Within the legal profession, definitions tend to focus on the documentation and investigation of a crime to determine culpability. It emphasizes the determination of guilt and innocence, applying laws and statutes and making decisions. Within the medical profession, definitions are composed largely on the basis of observable physiological consequences and effects of maltreatment or violence. In comparison, in mental health and social services, definitions focus on the familial setting, psychological consequences and effects, and the emphasis on determining the types of services to be provided. Definitions even differ within professions depending on the geographic region, and reflect variations in public, professional, and political opinions. Researchers struggle with the varying definitions since generalization of findings becomes difficult if different operational definitions are used from study to study. Those working with CEV often find communication difficult because of the definitional complexities. To date, there is not a standardized definition of CEV (Edmond, Fitzgerald, & Kracke, 2005; Mohr, Lutz, Fantuzzo, & Perry, 2000). In the present chapter and book, "children exposed to violence" will include *both* direct violence, such as child abuse, and indirect violence, such as growing up in a home with IPV or in a violent community (Office of Juvenile Justice and Delinquency Prevention, 2004; U.S. Department of Health and Human Services, Administration for Children and Families, 2005).

IMPACT OF CEV

The Adverse Childhood Experiences (ACE) study, a collaboration between the Centers for Disease Control and Prevention and Kaiser Permanente, demonstrated a link between child maltreatment and the most common causes of illness and death in America (Anda et al, 2006; Felitti et al., 1998). The key concept underlying the study is that stressful or traumatic childhood experiences intersect with social, emotional, and cognitive impairments that lead to increased risks of unhealthy behaviors, violence, polyvictimization, disease, disability, and premature death (Dube, Anda, Felitti, Edwards, & Williamson, 2002). Adverse childhood experiences can include: emotional, physical, and sexual abuse; emotional and physical neglect; exposure to IPV; and growing up with substance abusing or mentally ill household members.

Children of parents with a history of violence have an increased risk of exposure to violence themselves (Osofsky, 2004). Adults with a history of violence have been shown to be more likely to have a partner who is violent and to experience IPV (Anda et al., 2006; DeBellis, 2005; Widom & Maxfield, 1996). Children who are exposed to maltreatment or IPV also appear to be at greater risk for subsequent victimization (Daro, Edleson, & Pinderhughes, 2004). This has been referred to as polyvictimization (Finkelhor, Ormrod, & Turner, 2007).

Children's exposure to violence is also a major factor for later criminal behavior. For example, Widom (1989) found that child maltreatment increased the risk of overall arrests by 55% and arrests for a violent crime by 96%. Her study also revealed that, compared to a control group, maltreated children had an earlier onset of juvenile crime, more arrests, higher recidivism rates, and higher chronic offending. Maltreated children were nearly five times more likely to be arrested in their juvenile years and 11 times more likely to be arrested for violent crimes (Widom & Maxfield, 2001). Being abused or neglected as a child increased the likelihood of arrest as a juvenile by 53% and of arrest for a violent crime as an adult by 38% (OJJDP, 2004; Scowyra & Cocozza, 2007).

Recently, researchers have increasingly given attention to the effects of maltreatment and exposure to violence on the developing brain (e.g., Beers & DeBellis, 2002; Perry, 2001; Schonkoff & Phillips, 2000; Stien & Kendall, 2004). Developmental traumatology is the connection of the psychiatric and psychobiological fields when investigating the impact of violence on the developing child (Beers & DeBellis, 2002; DeBellis, 2005). An important directive of developmental traumatology is to make ecologically sound connections between a child's genetic constitution, critical and sensitive periods, psychosocial and cultural environment, and the influence that exposure to violence has had on the biological stress systems, brain development, and other known consequences (DeBellis, 2005; Perry, 2001).

Children's exposure to violence and trauma produce neurobiological impacts on the developing brain, including dysfunction in the hippocampus, amygdala, medial prefrontal cortex, and other limbic structures. When confronted with danger, the brain moves from an "information-processing" state to a survival-oriented, reactive "alarm state" (van der Kolk, Crozier, & Hopper, 2001). The relationship between CEV and later biopsychosocial development and functioning is complex, dynamic, and multi-layered. The dynamics of the neurophysiological responses of adults exposed to violence as children are discussed in more detail by Stride et al. (this book), with findings indicating that the situation is indeed complex. Systems that respond to CEV must be equally dynamic, as presented in the models described in this book (Becker et al.; Hyde et al.; Kracke & Cohen). Some of these are based on the Safe from the Start Initiative (OJJDP, 2000).

In order to advance the field of understanding CEV, it is important to identify the gaps and needs in different areas, as well as to suggest recommendations for overcoming the barriers and moving forward. The gaps and needs identified at the Think Tank are described below.

PRACTICE GAPS AND NEEDS

Practice Gaps

The practice gaps that were given high priority at the Think Tank fell into four categories. These included practice techniques, research-based practice, ecological framework, and screening/assessment.

1. Practice techniques
   - Public awareness of CEV is limited.
   - The current infrastructure is not prepared to be child-centered and family- and community-focused; there are no standard procedures for CEV (e.g., organized systems are not in place to deal with referrals).
   - The stigma associated with violence, abuse, and trauma may prevent individuals from seeking help.
   - The impact of violence on infants and very young children is often overlooked.
   - Primary, secondary, and tertiary prevention are not usually considered.
   - Despite the fact that multiple issues impact CEV, practice techniques continue to focus on and emphasize single factor solutions.
   - Practice techniques are not accessible to families that most need the information or are not available to professionals working with the most difficult-to-reach families.
   - Family preservation efforts and support funds are not consistently available.
2. Research-based practice
   - There is not yet a commitment to developing evidence-based practice, as well as to utilizing it and translating these practices into other domains.

- There usually is not an ongoing evaluation of the practice techniques utilized.
- Frontline providers are frequently unaware of current research, journals, reports, and books that are available on the subject.

3. Ecological framework
   - There is little effort to look at the child, family, community, and society collectively.
   - There is little fluidity of the systems interacting across a continuum or in a collaborative manner.
   - Consumer-survivors and nontraditional systems are not consistently included.

4. Screening and assessment
   - Screening tools are not available at all levels of practice within the community, and frontline practitioners do not usually emphasize assessment.
   - There are few screening efforts for prevention (e.g., screenings for risk factors or "red flags").
   - There is a lack of consistent, multi-disciplinary types of screening and assessment tools for CEV.
   - Screening and assessment measures and tools are not usually available to assess chronic and polyvictimization.

Practice Needs and Recommendations

There were a variety of practice needs identified at the Think Tank, and recommendations for dealing with them were suggested by those who worked on this topic. These were again divided into the same four categories listed above, and include:

1. Practice techniques
   - Social marketing techniques, such as those used to promote seatbelt use and smoking prevention, might be used to describe CEV as a public health problem.
   - Building a collective sense of responsibility for children and engaging the public in a discussion about how the prevalence and impact of CEV would be powerful components of a long-term strategy to prevent and reduce CEV.
   - Prior to a campaign, a social cost analysis needs to be performed to attest to the need of such a campaign. To accurately reflect the impact for such a campaign, it is essential to have the most recent

data on the incidence and prevalence of CEV (see chapter by Kracke & Hahn, this book).

- Research continues to show the significant neurological impacts of violence on the developing; therefore, practice techniques must evolve by integrating new research on the impact of exposure to violence on neurodevelopment.
- Two practice issues that need to be addressed are system structure and system engagement as they relate to CEV within various systems of community care.

2. Research-based practice
   - Federal support is needed to sustain research and dissemination. Federal agencies must make a commitment to evaluating promising approaches and developing evidence-based practices. This commitment must be reinforced at the state and local levels to ensure that promising practices are not eliminated because the outcome evidence has not yet been obtained with evaluation studies.
   - Research in the area of practice should be encouraged in order to build knowledge and improve effectiveness of intervention programs.
   - It is helpful for more practitioners to engage in research with researchers, and for researchers to work with practitioners to evaluate practice. Furthermore, fidelity and flexibility in practice should be encouraged across systems and individuals.
   - The cultural implications of practice should be considered when conducting practice and outcome research.
   - The core set of standards in terms of utilizing evidence-based practice should be defined but flexible, and practitioners should receive professional development in order to be able to identify appropriate strategies to implement them effectively.
   - Research findings need to be presented in clear and practical language, perhaps jargon-free, for the benefit of practitioners and community members.
   - Agencies that base program development upon research findings need to continuously observe and evaluate the practice techniques, gathering data on satisfaction and efficacy among families served.
   - Incentives could be provided to agencies that continuously incorporate evaluation into practice, and a percentage of all funding for intervention and prevention programs should be for the evaluation of effectiveness.

- Dissemination of research findings needs to be timely, consistent, accurate, and targeted to every system associated with CEV. For example, professionals in the field need training on evidence-based practices as they are established, and they need training manuals that are translated, targeted to the audience, and with the ecological framework embedded.
- Those practitioners accessing the training information should be provided with sustained technical assistance after the training is complete.

3. Ecological framework
   - Cross-system processes must be defined through open dialogue among professionals working in all areas of CEV. Although there are unique components important to individual agencies, there should also be a convergence across systems that respond to CEV.
   - From an ecological framework, the systems of care should be more than child-centered; they would also include family, community, and social factors. A part of an ecological framework would include an understanding of how the child's ecology is relevant to each system.
   - The system of care should be multi-disciplinary, interconnected, seamless, and include nontraditional influences.

4. Screening and assessment
   - Professionals and community members need a better understanding of CEV and the etiology, signs, symptoms, ramifications, and behavioral manifestations grounded in research and evidence-based practice. First responders, including firefighters, police, members of the medical community, child welfare workers, educators, and members of faith- and community-based organizations, have the opportunity to recognize a potential problem and refer the family for help.
   - The agencies responsible for CEV could benefit from learning about risk factors and screening. These systems also need to interact and collaborate with one another for a continuum of care.
   - Professionals in all related fields, community members, and consumer-survivors need to come together and restructure the systems of care so that no child or family falls through the identified gaps of the current systems. Screening and assessment are key aspects of this process.
   - There needs to be identified referral paths for each system so that the professionals and community members know where victims of CEV can find various forms of assistance.

- Better assessment tools are needed to help identify a range of issues across ages and developmental stages.
- Assessment tools should be incorporated across disciplines. The selection of clinical instruments affects outcomes and treatments, so it is important to develop reliable and standardized tools and measures that embrace the diverse components of cultures and incorporate an understanding of those families that are often over-represented but underserved in the various systems.
- The next step is to define specific identification mechanisms for each system in order to get children to the right place at the right time.
- It is necessary to promote more consistent, multi-disciplinary types of screening and to build better knowledge about formal screening identification assessments.

TRAINING GAPS AND NEEDS

Training Gaps

Three categories of training gaps were identified at the Think Tank: Content and Process, the Audience, and Evaluation and Technical Assistance.

1. Content and process
   - The importance of training is not well understood by many agencies (i.e., it may be the first component of programs to be cut when funding is reduced).
   - Training goals are often unclear.
   - Trainers may not always have core knowledge of topics.
   - Methods for delivery of training may not be sufficiently diverse.
   - Adult learning techniques may not be used often.
   - Training is not always developed and delivered using a multi-disciplinary approach.
   - Most trainings do not incorporate the voices of children, victims, or survivors.
   - Training concerning trauma and CEV is not yet sufficiently incorporated into the curriculum of graduate and undergraduate institutions.
2. Audience
   - Much training is not geared to the specific audience.
   - Accountability for learned material is usually not evaluated or ensured by the training programs.

- The trainers usually do not have direct input by consumers and survivors to ensure that these perspectives are included and relevant.
- Broad and introductory training is often lacking for all those who are part of one or more systems of care.

3. Evaluation and technical assistance
   - Evaluations of training programs are often limited in their determination of the usefulness of the material and techniques and whether participants actually utilize the techniques.
   - Additional evaluation tools and alternative types of procedures are often lacking (e.g., internet and phone follow-up surveys).
   - There is often a lack of technical assistance once training is completed.

Training Needs and Recommendations

The following training needs and recommendations were identified by the Think Tank participants and are listed utilizing the same categories as noted above.

1. Content and process
   - Education and training are needed to change attitudes and behaviors. Training should be used to advance both knowledge and practice. It can also be instrumental in improving systems of care.
   - Agencies need to identify their goals and needs for training in conjunction with staff and clients. It is important for trainers to assess agencies prior to the trainings in order to identify potential barriers that may impede learning so that they can be considered to improve the training.
   - Trainers and agencies need to work together to be clear about the purpose of training and why training is needed. Learning objectives and outcomes also need to be defined; it should also be emphasized that training is only the first step in advancing knowledge and implementing changes.
   - There are core competencies that encompass a large range of issues that trainers need to have. The trainers should have knowledge and competencies in child and brain development and knowledge of systems and roles.
   - The training should be culturally relevant and tailored to the specific audience.
   - Trainers should have formal training about adult learning techniques.

- The content of the training should include the views and opinions of children, adult victims, trainees, the community, and the community's represented cultures. The training should be multi-disciplinary, and include an integrated, multi-level, and system-wide approach.
- There should be guidelines for strategic training and how to evaluate the training.
- It is also important that a clearinghouse for dissemination and the identified core competencies of each discipline be developed. It would be helpful to have a national inventory or clearinghouse of core components of training (e.g., child development, brain development, impact, and prevalence) in the areas of curriculum materials. These resources need to be easily accessible (e.g., via the web). These trainings should also be incorporated into universities and into the curriculum of graduate and undergraduate institutions.
- Mechanisms for communicating training is important and should include a creative continuum of methodology to deliver training that is easily accessible to its audience. For example, trainers could use distance learning, online interactive learning, major conferences, direct training, video, phone and conference calls, and on-site instruction as techniques to reach a large audience.
- Training is most effective when delivered immediately and proactively; thus, wide scale implementation is critical to garner benefits from competent training.

2. Audience
   - Identifying and recruiting an audience from traditional and nontraditional sources is important.
   - An ecological training approach may be the most effective approach. When agencies and communities come together to be trained, the knowledge exchanged will likely be beneficial for the children and families served.
   - The purpose of the training should be issues related to CEV and tailored to the needs and goals of the audience. The training should be expanded to include businesses (corporations and small businesses), coaches and team members, faith-based providers, new parents and people in parenting groups, schools at the undergraduate and graduate level, community leaders, and elected officials.

3. Evaluation and technical assistance
   - It is important for organizations to have a clear understanding of how they will be held accountable for maintaining a certain level

of training. The effectiveness of the training also needs to be evaluated by some measurable outcome.

- Training is only one of the strategies that need to be put in place in order to make concrete changes. Evaluation must be conducted to ascertain the effectiveness of trainings. The impact of trainings and overall impact of change in the trainees need to be measured. The training needs to be evaluated at the institution and system levels as well as at an individual level (i.e., participatory evaluations).
- An evaluation plan should be put in place that includes a way to assess behavior change resulting from the training (e.g., a 6-week follow up).
- Tools that can be utilized in the evaluation and delivery of training or services process include video, internet, proactive training, and phone consultation.
- Technical assistance and trainings should go hand-in-hand (i.e., training is an ongoing process that is enhanced by follow-up technical assistance).

RESEARCH AND EVALUATION GAPS AND NEEDS

The Think Tank participants identified three main categories of gaps in the research and evaluation of CEV: research standards, outcomes research, and dynamics of CEV research.

Research and Evaluation Gaps

1. Research standards
   - Definitions of terms are not consistent and different professions use similar terms to mean different behaviors.
   - The population studied is often not specified sufficiently, and diverse cultures are not always included in the research nor adequately understood.
   - Measurement scales and procedures are not often agreed upon (e.g., developmental stages and predictive validity of informants may not be adequately considered when designing measures).
   - Guidelines for a better way to synthesize multi-media informant data and multiple methods of obtaining data are not established for basic intervention and prevention research.
   - Mandated reporting may skew research and challenge the integrity of the data.

- Guidelines are often lacking for community research partnerships and advisory boards to develop CEV tools and products for granters, grantees, and researchers.
- Foundations and granters may not have adequate knowledge or expertise on research methodology.

2. Outcome research
- Chronological age at time of trauma, proximity, severity, and frequency of trauma are not usually considered when observing externalized behaviors, including aggression, delinquent behaviors, conduct problems, and academic performance.
- Tools are lacking to improve the speed with which data are collected in order to reduce the disparity between research and practice.
- Research information is often not translated well from one discipline to another, or to those on the front lines and at the community level.
- There are inconsistent dissemination standards (i.e., professional journals vs. literature for the lay public). The community cannot utilize the research if they do not have access to it or understand it.

3. Dynamics of CEV research
- At times there appears to be a disconnect between those conducting the research and those who are the recipients of the research.
- A gap exists between prevention and intervention research.
- Families involved in court cases are an infrequently studied population for intervention efforts, and are thus often absent from the literature; we do not know whether these people are systematically different from the groups studied or whether they experience the same dynamics.

Research and Evaluation Needs and Recommendations

1. Research standards:
- Multiple systems and community members need to come together to establish guidelines for quality of research, data collection, and common psychometrics. Issues of concern include fidelity, protocol adherence, dissemination of findings, misuse of data, and translation of research into jargon-free language.
- Research needs to be multidisciplinary and the inclusion of consumer survivors in the design of the study should guide its

formulation, recruitment of research participants, evaluation, dissemination, and education.

- Definitions also need to be collaboratively developed by researchers with input from those who have been exposed to violence and are involved in the systems of care. Definitions need to address types of abuse, cultural influences, relevant laws, the target population, and mediating and moderating factors.
- It is important to decide how to use measurement scales and the appropriateness of the scales for the research. There is also a challenge in designing evaluations that are sensitive to and that catch the subtle differences of individuals.
- Many scales and questionnaires are limited because of language differences, communication difficulties, and problems with adaptation to different populations. Therefore, multicultural, developmental, and biopsychosocial issues must be considered in the development and implementation of assessment tools.
- Although mandated reporting is necessary, the consequences of such reporting create a challenge to conducting research. The ethical dilemmas involved in asking parents known to be involved in violence and abuse to join research projects need to be resolved with solutions provided (ideally to include the parent before maltreatment has occurred). Those participating in research should be educated about the relevant laws and policies regarding mandated reporting for types of violence. Confidentiality issues should be reviewed.

2. Outcome research
   - Researchers or evaluators need to involve practitioners and consumer survivors in the design and implementation of outcome research. The interpretation of the results of the research and the translation of the findings into practice are enhanced and more meaningful when ecological context is considered. Research must be translated in a way such that those impacted by CEV can make use of it.
   - Research needs to be fluid as knowledge in the field and the dynamics of the research studies change (e.g., will the modifiable research and evaluation, based on systems needs, affect outcome?).
   - Identifying the most proximal mediators and modifiable factors, including stressors, problems, and parenting practices, is important. In terms of trauma exposure, it is important to consider temporal issues, especially when working with children and families. Research and evaluation must be trauma-informed.

- Research needs to be better utilized to inform clinical practice and policy standards as opposed to primarily for academic publication status. Research can be used to empower and engage systems and community members.
3. Dynamics of CEV
   - Recognition of different areas of violence should be addressed (e.g., not only IPV but also other traumatic experiences, such as community violence). Exposure to violence has many levels (threat, physical violence, acute and chronic violence) and research is needed on exposure to differing levels of violence.
   - Fostering an understanding between researchers and consumers of research is needed. Community education on best practice interventions should be conducted in order to imbed them into practice and into the structure of the community.
   - Attaining valid and reliable data is another challenge. Tools need to be developed that not only provide insights for these situations (e.g., outcomes, effectiveness, and consequences) but also for the etiology.
   - There are also political issues that can hinder research. Because of child welfare issues, researchers and administrators may feel threatened by outcome findings that negatively impinge on their agency or program. Furthermore, due to the liability and confidential nature of the courts, there is not as much research conducted in court settings as is needed.

POLICY GAPS AND NEEDS

The Think Tank also focused on policy gaps and needs. Participants identified three main priority categories in the policy arena for CEV. These are reactive versus proactive systems, fragmented systems, and social policy supporting systems integration versus systems abuse.

Policy Gaps

1. Reactive vs. proactive systems
   - A focus on critical incident response results in isolation and a lack of attention to fundamental issues.
   - Child death review committees may address some of the issues of CEV, as it often takes a tragedy or death to initiate or focus on the issues of violence.

- Red flags and risk factors are not currently addressed. People do not recognize red flags that exist, and often there are no services to provide when they are noted.
- Breaking up the family is sometimes provided as the answer, but often this is not effective because displaced family members often continue the relationship in the future or atleast continue contact.

2. Fragmented systems
   - Fragmentation of the systems is often the status quo (e.g., only parts of the issue, like substance abuse, may be addressed).
   - There is a system's problem when families in need of assistance are not identified and families perceive that professionals do not care about them or their issues.
   - There are problems with the language of statutes and definitions, and many people do not have an adequate understanding of what the statutes mean.

3. Social policy supporting systems integration vs. systems abuse
   - Legislation and policy was originally based on the child victims of abuse, and not the family from an ecological perspective.
   - Legislation and policy, and therefore interventions, were often based on punitive action that did not take into account the full scope of the issues.
   - The legal system has not been adequately updated to deal with the complex issues of violence within the family.
   - Child welfare systems often respond only after critical incidents have occurred.
   - Too often the legal and social services systems rely on the notion that the child is the sole person affected by violence. This notion leads to child removal, which may not be effective as a solution to CEV.
   - A public health model is not nationally utilized.
   - There are few national prevention or intervention efforts for parents on how to be healthy parents.

Policy Needs and Recommendations

1. Reactive vs. proactive systems
   - To fill the gaps between reaction and prevention strategies, a commitment needs to be made at the national level to make funding available for prevention efforts. The flexibility of the use of those funds can be transferred to the state and local county agencies familiar with local needs. This investment, if made in the early

years of the child's development, can have lasting impacts over the course of the child's life. This is an example of an economic strategy that invests in the system at the front end rather than paying for the cost of violence after it has occurred.

- Two systems are needed: the current reactive system that responds when an incident occurs and a system that works to prevent violence. For example, by way of secondary intervention, Child Welfare Services could reach out to a family in need of help and provide a voluntary system for families. Ideally, prevention efforts would include all members of the family and the intervention would happen before violence occurs; in reactive systems, these same individuals are sometimes identified as victims or perpetrators.
- A public health and multidisciplinary team approach should be utilized in primary prevention efforts. Embracing this approach, professional cross-training and community forums are needed to address the identified issues surrounding youth at-risk for exposure to violence (e.g., developmental psychology, developmental psychopathology, substance abuse, IPV, and neurodevelopment).

2. Fragmented systems
   - The policy system needs to be flexible in its treatment of adults. Perhaps some of the tension that exists surrounding the disclosure of IPV would be reduced or eliminated if systems were not competing for scarce resources, especially funding.
   - Dynamic policy and funding streams need to be developed for programs that work best for children and families. These programs must also evolve as the needs of the community change and as knowledge continues to grow in the field.
   - Policies and prevention efforts should be family and ecologically centered. A collective concern for children may be the most effective way to engage families.
   - Individual differences and strengths of the child and family should be addressed, including risk and protective factors and cultural and societal norms. For instance, recent research on ACEs, the brain, and neurodevelopment appears to be effective in increasing awareness. Therefore, it is pertinent that policies include funding to facilitate neurological assessments of the needs of a child who has been exposed to chronic trauma. With this information, practitioners may redirect techniques according

to the results (e.g., move from usual cognitive behavioral therapy techniques to trauma-focused cognitive behavioral therapy).

- Policymakers, legislative leaders, researchers, practitioners, advocates, and funders need to come together to become more familiar with the various systems of care and the unique needs and strengths of each system. Thus, policies need to rely very little on one size fits all approaches and more on the distinct ecology of the family system as it relates to available systems of care.

3. Social policy supporting systems integration vs. systems abuse
   - Uniform national definitions are needed. With separate definitions, systems cannot communicate as effectively, and research findings are not generalizeable.
   - Within the consumer-survivor movement, currently supported by the Substance Abuse and Mental Health Services Administration, the statement that informs policy is: "Nothing about us, without us." It is difficult to understand the dynamics concerning an individual's life experiences without his/her unique interpretation. If the systems of care are not capturing or understanding the clients' experiences accurately, the outcome may not be productive.
   - Child-centered policy should be created within the ecological and family system. The needs of the child are paramount, and there should be a way to engage parents in a voluntary commitment to action.
   - A specific timeframe for interventions should be in place for working with parents when children are born. Prevention programs must be given a greater emphasis and should be nonpunitive, culturally specific, and sensitive to the needs of the family. The systems that are already in use are difficult to restructure.
   - A social and public health marketing campaign for CEV should be developed (e.g., "Market Healthy Children"). The idea should be to invest in a product that will become a tool for primary prevention, which should include producing healthy families and not in repairing what is broken. It is crucial to reach out to the Advertising Council in such a marketing campaign.

CONCLUSION AND IMPLICATIONS FOR CHILDREN, FAMILIES, AND SYSTEMS OF CARE

The Think Tank breakout groups focused overall on issues, gaps, and recommendations for CEV and their families. In summary, seven major issues were identified. These include:

1. CEV needs to be recognized as a public health problem.
2. Child development, including neurodevelopment, should be integrated into all aspects of research, policy, practice, evaluation, assessment, and training.
3. Prevention and intervention efforts must be child-centered within the family context.
4. Embracing a multidisciplinary and ecologically sound approach would enhance systems of care for children and families.
5. A tiered approach (from frontline workers to supervisors to community members) enhances prevention and intervention efforts.
6. CEV needs a coordinated and multidisciplinary marketing campaign.
7. A guide for strategic planning for systems and communities needs to be developed.

The current system in place for CEV is predominately reactive. When systems are fragmented, barriers may develop that can disable coordination among agencies. Barriers can consist of a lack of understanding of contrasting policies and procedures, competing visions, variations in roles, a lack of trust between individuals from different agencies, and insufficient resources to facilitate collaboration. Despite this, some individuals within a system take it upon themselves to initiate informal collaboration due to the perceived benefits that accompany joint investigations and information-sharing. Without continued endorsement and commitment to collaboration on the part of agency leaders, those who are at other levels within the institution may hold different views and, consequently, inhibit the effectiveness of collaboration.

When systems are reactive versus proactive, policies and procedures may develop to lessen the burden on the system, but may be counterproductive overall. For instance, the child welfare screening process was developed across the social services systems in an effort to manage the increasing number of suspected child maltreatment cases. As a result, agencies and states adopted more restrictive definitions of abuse, thus limiting the number of intakes or investigations. The screening process, although focusing investigations on the most serious allegations, may actually further the risk of children and families who have been screened out because they did not evidence the most serious incidents at the time. Therefore, an incident that is not substantiated does not necessarily mean that the child and family are at a lower risk for future maltreatment or that maltreatment did not occur.

We can no longer approach any social issue from a singular lens, as isolated agencies, nor can we continue the vertical projection of research, training, policy, and practice. To do so would cause more harm than good. Steps have been made to improve research, training, policy, and practice (e.g., 42 states and the District of Columbia recognized that children who are exposed to violence need to be protected from the emotional abuse that ensues from the IPV exposure; U.S. Department of Health and Human Services, 2005). This is the first step, but more follow-up and additional steps are needed to actually intervene in these cases or to prevent such abuse. When there is a collective commitment and shared responsibility, a system can then begin to build the type of changes that include reciprocity and mutual support, thus creating an opportunity to make lasting changes in children's lives. It is hoped that the chapters in this book provide greater awareness of the issues involved with CEV, stimulate additional research, improve practice techniques, lead to more evidence-based programs for both intervention as well as prevention, and help initiate a national priority to eliminate violence in the home and community.

REFERENCES

Anda, R. F., Felitti, V.J., Walker, J., Whitfield, C. L., Bremner, J. D., Perry, B. D., et al. (2006). The enduring effects of abuse and related adverse experiences in childhood: A convergence of evidence from neurobiology and epidemiology. *European Archives of Psychiatry and Clinical Neurosciences, 56*(3), 174–186.

Beers, S., & De Bellis, M. (2002). Neuropsychological function in children with maltreatment-related posttraumatic stress disorder. *American Journal of Psychiatry, 159*, 483–486.

Daro, D., Edleson, J. L., & Pinderhughes, H. (2004). Finding common ground in the study of child maltreatment, youth violence, and adult domestic violence. *Journal of Interpersonal Violence, 19*(3), 282–298.

De Bellis, M. D. (2005). The psychobiology of neglect. *Child Maltreatment, 10*, 150–172.

Dube, S. R., Anda, R. F., Felitti, V. J., Edwards, V., & Williamson, D. F. (2002). Exposure to abuse, neglect and household dysfunction among adults who witnessed intimate partner violence as children. *Violence and Victims, 17*(1), 3–17.

Edmond, Y., Fitzgerald, M., & Kracke, K. (2005). *Incidence and prevalence of children exposed to violence: A research review.* Unpublished manuscript available from authors at Office of Juvenile Justice and Delinquency Prevention (OJJDP), U.S. Department of Justice, Washington, DC.

Felitti, V. J., Anda, R. F., Nordenberg, D., Williamson, D. F., Spitz, A. M., Edwards, V., et al. (1998). Relationship of childhood abuse and household dysfunction to many of the leading causes of death in adults: The Adverse Childhood Experiences (ACE) Study. *American Journal of Preventive Medicine, 14*(4), 245–258.

Finkelhor, D., Ormrod, R., & Turner H. (2007). Poly-victimization: A neglected component in child victimization. *Child Abuse and Neglect, 31*, 7–26.

Geffner, R., Igelman, R. S., & Zellner, J. (Eds.) (2003). *Effects of intimate partner violence on children.* Binghamton, NY: Haworth Maltreatment & Trauma Press.

Geffner, R. A., Jaffe, P. G., & Sudermann, M. (Eds.). (2000). *Children exposed to domestic violence: Current issues in research, intervention, prevention, and policy development.* Binghamton, NY: Haworth Maltreatment & Trauma Press.

Geffner, R., & Rosenbaum, A. (2002). Domestic violence offenders: Treatment and intervention standards. In R. Geffner & A. Rosenbaum (Eds.), *Domestic violence offenders: Current interventions, research, and implications for policies and standards* (pp. 1–9). Binghamton, NY: Haworth Maltreatment & Trauma Press.

Groves, B. M., Augustyn, M., Lee, D., & Sawires, P. (2002). *Identifying and responding to domestic violence: Consensus recommendations for child and adolescent health.* San Francisco, CA: Family Violence Prevention Fund.

Mohr, W. K., Lutz, M. J. N., Fantuzzo, J. W., & Perry, M. A. (2000). Children exposed to family violence: A review of empirical research from a developmental-ecological perspective. *Trauma, Violence, & Abuse, 1*(3), 264–283.

Office of Juvenile Justice and Delinquency Prevention (OJJDP). (2000, November). *Safe from the start: Taking action on children exposed to violence.* Publication No. NCJ182789. Washington, DC: U.S. Department of Justice, Office of Justice Programs.

Office of Juvenile Justice and Delinquency Prevention (OJJDP) (2004). *Statistical briefing book.* Washington, DC: U.S. Department of Justice, Office of Justice Programs.

Osofsky, J. (Ed.) (2004). *Young children and trauma: Intervention and treatment.* New York: Guilford Publications.

Perry, B. D. (2001). The neuroarcheology of child maltreatment: The neurodevelopmental costs of adverse childhood events. In K. Franey, R. Geffner, & R. Falconer (Eds.), *The cost of child maltreatment: Who pays? We all do* (pp. 15–37). San Diego, CA: Family Violence & Sexual Assault Institute.

Schonkoff, J. P., & Phillips, D. A. (2000). *From neurons to neighborhoods: The science of early childhood development.* Washington, DC: National Academy Press.

Scowyra, K. R., & Cocozza, J. J. (2007). *Blueprint for change: A comprehensive model for the identification and treatment of youth with mental health needs in contact with the juvenile justice system.* National Center for Mental Health and Juvenile Justice, Office of Juvenile Justice and Delinquency Prevention, U.S., Department of Justice Report. Delmar, NY: Policy Research Associates, Inc.

Stien, P. T., & Kendall, J. (2004). *Psychological trauma and the developing brain: Neurologically based interventions for troubled children.* Binghamton, NY: Haworth Maltreatment & Trauma Press.

Stith, S. M., Smith, D. B., Penn, C. E., Ward, D. B., & Tritt, D. (2004). Intimate partner physical abuse perpetration and victimization risk factors: A meta-analytic review. *Aggression and Violent Behavior, 10,* 65–98.

U.S. Department of Health and Human Services, Administration for Children and Families. (2005). *Child maltreatment 2003.* Washington, DC: U.S. Government Printing Office.

van der Kolk, B. A., Crozier, J., & Hopper, J. (2001). Child abuse in America: Prevalence, costs, consequences, and intervention. In K. Franey, R. Geffner, & R. Falconer (Eds.), *The cost of child maltreatment: Who pays? We all do* (pp. 223–241). San Diego, CA: Family Violence & Sexual Assault Institute.

Widom, C. S. (1989). Child abuse, neglect, and adult behavior: Research design and findings on criminality, violence, and child abuse. *American Journal of Orthopsychiatry, 59,* 355–367.

Widom, C. S., & Maxfield, M. G. (1996). Cycle of violence: Revisited six years later. *Archives of Pediatrics and Adolescent Medicine, 150,* 390–395.

Widom, C. S., & Maxfield, M. G. (2001). *An update on the "cycle of violence."* Washington, DC: U.S. Department of Justice, Office of Justice Programs, National Institute of Justice NCJ 184894.

APPENDIX

Think Tank Participants and Their Affiliations

Bailey, Christine, JD, Director of Permanency Planning for Children, National Council of Juvenile and Family Court Judges, Reno, NV

Chamberlain, Linda, PhD, Founding Director, Alaska Family Violence Prevention Project, Anchorage, AK

Cohen, Elena P., Director of the Safe Start Center at JBS International, Silver Spring, MD

da Silva, Julia, MA, Director, Office of Violence Prevention, American Psychological Association, Washington, DC

Deserly, Kathy, President, Indian Child and Family Resource Center, Helena, MT

Diesman, Kathleen, MEd, JD, Deputy District Attorney, Los Angeles District Attorney's Office, Long Beach, CA

Geffner, Robert, PhD, President, Institute on Violence, Abuse and Trauma at Alliant International University, San Diego, CA

Gewirtz, Abigail, PhD, University of Minnesota, Minneapolis, MN

Griffin, Dawn Alley, PhD, Alliant International University, San Diego, CA

Harrington, Roy, MS, Project Director, Spokane's Safe Start Initiative, WA

Holton, John, PhD, Vice President for Research, Prevent Child Abuse, America, Chicago, IL

Hyde, Mary Morris, PhD, Senior Managing Associate, Association for the Study and Development of Community, Gaithersburg, MD

Imagawa, Karen, MD, Children's Hospital, Los Angeles, CA

Jaycox, Lisa, PhD, Senior Behavioral Scientist, Rand Corporation, Washington, DC

Johnson, Deborah, MA, Director of National Services, Children's Institute, Rochester, NY

Kracke, Kristen, MSW, Safe Start Initiative Coordinator and Program Manager, Office of Juvenile Justice and Delinquency Prevention, Washington, DC

Lederman, Cindy, JD, Administrative Judge of the Juvenile Division Juvenile Justice Center, 11th Judicial Circuit - State of Florida, Miami

Leeb, Rebecca, PhD, Division of Violence Prevention, Centers for Disease Control and Prevention, Atlanta, GA

Levenson, Rebecca, MA, Senior Health Associate, Family Violence Prevention Fund, San Francisco, CA

Lewis III, James, PsyD, Chief Operating Officer, National Center on Children Exposed to Violence at the Yale Child Study Center, New Haven, CT

McAlister-Groves, Betsy, MSW, Director, Child Witness to Violence Project, Boston, MA

McDonald, Renee, PhD, Family Research Center, Southern Methodist University, Dallas, TX

Melmed, Matthew, JD, Executive Director Zero to Three, National Center for Infants, Toddlers and Families, Washington, DC

Rosenbaum, Alan, PhD, Department of Psychology, Northern Illinois University, DeKalb, IL

Simpson, Judith, MBA, Program Manager, Pinellas Safe Start, Juvenile Welfare Board of Pinellas, FL

Van Horn, Patricia, JD, PhD, Child Trauma Research Project, San Francisco General Hospital,

White, Marlita, LCSW, Director, Chicago Safe Start, Office of Violence Prevention, Department of Public Health, IL

Wong-Kerberg, Linda, LMFT, Director, Office of Violence Prevention, County of San Diego Health and Human Services, CA

The Nature and Extent of Childhood Exposure to Violence: What We Know, Why We Don't Know More, and Why It Matters

Kristen Kracke
Hilary Hahn

Children in the United States are exposed to violence in alarming numbers. Estimates for children's exposure to violence vary widely from 3.3 million to 10 million to 17 million (Carlson, 1984; Holden, 1998; Silvern et al., 1995; Straus, 1991). These numbers are often presented as our best effort to quantify children's exposure to violence in general, but actually refer to one subset of violence exposure: children that witness domestic violence. These numbers do not count violence that is inflicted upon children directly or violence that children experience outside their homes. Nonetheless, this picture of children's welfare is disheartening and has generated significant concern among a broad range of professionals, policymakers, and service providers, including medical and health professionals, child protection and social services agencies, intimate partner violence (IPV) service providers, and advocates, law enforcement, and juvenile justice agencies. However, while estimates of various forms of exposure to violence suggest that the problem is persistent and insidious and that action to address the problem is needed, the active and growing multidisciplinary concern about childhood exposure to violence (CEV) has developed in advance of concrete information documenting the full extent and nature of the problem. Childhood exposure to violence data is limited by the historical tendency of researchers and practitioners to define the problem by type of exposure, and existing data is likely to significantly underestimate the magnitude of the problem. This article presents information currently available on the nature and extent of CEV, identifies some critical gaps in the knowledge base, discusses key challenges to developing a comprehensive picture of the CEV problem, and presents recommendations intended to address these challenges and serve the needs of researchers and practitioners alike.

WHAT IS KNOWN ABOUT THE NATURE AND EXTENT OF CHILDHOOD EXPOSURE TO VIOLENCE?

Data on CEV comes from a variety of sources, including official crime data surveys, public health epidemiological studies, and social science research (Frierson, 1999), most of which categorize CEV into varying loci such as violence at home, in the community, or at school. There have been relatively few studies designed to explore or quantify children's total exposure to violence. Two recent relevant efforts to develop a comprehensive account of the problem of CEV are the Adverse Childhood Experiences (ACE) Study (Centers for Disease Control and Prevention [CDC], 2006a; Felitti et al., 1998) and the Developmental Victimization Survey (DVS; Finkelhor, Ormrod, Turner, & Hamby, 2005). Co-sponsored by the CDC, the ACE Study is one of the largest investigations ever conducted on the links between childhood adversity and later-life health and well-being. It is a retrospective study of more than 17,000 members of the Kaiser Permanente health maintenance organization and examined seven categories of ACEd. The number of ACE categories was then compared to measures of adult risk behavior, health status, and disease. Almost two-thirds of study participants reported at least one ACE, and more than 1 in 5 reported three or more. The short- and long-term outcomes of these childhood exposures include a multitude of health and social problems in later childhood, adolescence, and adulthood that are compounded with the number of ACE reported (CDC, 2006a; Felitti et al., 1998). While the ACE Study does not provide specific incidence and prevalence rates of CEV, it does indicate that the problem's extent and consequences are significant.

The DVS, conducted in 2003 by University of New Hampshire using the Juvenile Victimization Questionnaire (JVQ), obtained 1-year incidence estimates of a comprehensive range of childhood victimizations across gender, race, and developmental stage. Administered to a nationally representative sample of 1000 children aged 10 to 17 and 1030 caregivers of children aged 2 to 9 living in the United States, the JVQ gathered reports on 34 forms of offenses against youth covering five general areas of concern: conventional crime, child maltreatment, peer and sibling victimization, sexual assault, and witnessing and indirect victimization (Finkelhor et al., 2005). They found that child maltreatment occurred to a little more than 1 in 7 of the child and youth population (138 per 1000). One-third (357 per 1000) of the national sample of children and youth had witnessed the victimization of another person or been exposed to victimization indirectly in the course of the study year. Among the 71% of all children and youth who reported at least one direct or indirect victimization, the average juvenile victim was victimized in three different ways in separate incidents during the course of a year. Children and youth with any sexual victimization were particularly likely (97%) to have additional victimizations, especially an assault (82%) or a witnessing or indirect victimization (84%).

In comparison to previous victimization studies such as the National Crime Victimization Survey, the estimates of specific types of victimization in the DVS are generally higher. For a variety of victimizations such as bias attacks, bullying, and witnessing physical abuse, the DVS provides the first national estimates from a population survey. In addition, the DVS provides victimization estimates across the full age range of childhood, a study feature seldom available. Further enhancement of the DVS data is needed to specifically capture the full nature and extent of CEV, particularly in the subtype area of witnessing partner violence. In addition, more detailed information about the type, frequency, intensity, proximity, location, and victim/perpetrator relationship in areas of indirect victimization would be beneficial. These enhancements of the DVS are currently underway and are discussed below; however, the DVS clearly indicates that considerable CEV is masked by such limitations.

The ACE and DVS studies are unusual in their attempt to document the full nature and extent of CEV. More commonly, CEV studies and data sets provide estimates of the incidence and prevalence of specific types of CEV, such as witnessing domestic violence. As a result, we must look at what is currently known in these separate types of exposure: child maltreatment, IPV, community violence, and school violence. While child maltreatment is often not included in discussions of CEV, child maltreatment is included here because it represents the most direct form of violence and is essential for developing a complete understanding of the violence that children in this country experience in their daily lives. Furthermore, the level of co-occurrence and multiple victimizations is high and underscores the importance of a comprehensive and inclusive definition of CEV. Stratifying exposure data according to the location of the event, the "primary" victim, or characteristics of the offender presents significant difficulties to researchers, practitioners, and policymakers, failing to acknowledge the potential cumulative impacts of events and the compounding effects of multiple exposures. However, at this time, these studies are essential to our understanding of CEV.

Child Maltreatment: Incidence and Prevalence

The U.S. Department of Health and Human Services (HHS) collects data annually from state child protective services agencies through the National Child Abuse and Neglect Data System (NCANDS). In 2005, an estimated 899,000 children nationwide were identified as victims of abuse and neglect from substantiated cases in the child welfare system. Because this figure counts only substantiated cases, the numbers are largely underrepresentative of the problem of direct child maltreatment. Of these substantiated cases, though, the number represents a victimization rate of 12.1 per 1000 children. More than half of these victims (62.8%) experienced neglect, while 16.6% were physically abused, 9.3% were sexually abused, and 7.1% were emotionally or psychologically maltreated. The rate of victimization was inversely related to the age of the child: children age 3 and younger accounted for the highest rate of victimization and children ages 7 and younger accounted for 54.5% of all child victims (Children's Bureau, 2005a). In addition, researchers have found that the severity of child victimization is greater for children younger than age 5 (Dilillo, Tremblay, & Peterson, 2000).

The NCANDS also documented in 2005 that approximately 6.0 million children were alleged to be maltreated through an estimated 3.3 million referrals to Child Protective Services (CPS) agencies (more than half of which were made by professionals; Children's Bureau, 2005a). These numbers represent only those children known to the CPS agencies and must therefore be considered "the tip of the iceberg" as indicated by the National Incidence Study (NIS) of Child Abuse and Neglect, which is currently conducting data collection for NIS-4 (Children's Bureau, 2005b). NIS-3, conducted in 1993, provides the most current available data and highlights that an estimated 1.5 million children were abused or neglected, which reflected a 67% increase since the NIS-2 estimate in 1986 (Sedlak & Broadhurst, 1996).

Intimate Partner Violence: Incidence and Prevalence

Data from the National Violence Against Women Survey indicates that 5.3 million intimate partner victimizations of women over age 18 occur in the United States each year, resulting in 2 million injuries (CDC, 2003). Nonfatal intimate partner victimization for females was about 4 victimizations per 1000 persons age 12 and older in 2004 (Catalano, 2006). While the number of intimate partner homicide victims has declined since

1993 from 1571 females murdered in 1993 to 1159 during 2004 (Catalano, 2006), it is clear that IPV is a significant risk factor for various physical and mental health problems and is one of the most common causes of injury in women (Rennison & Rand, 2003).

Estimates from the National Crime Victimization Survey indicate that during 2004 there were approximately 627,400 nonfatal intimate partner victimizations and that children resided in 43% of the households in which IPV occurred with a female victim (Catalano, 2006). Findings from the Spousal Assault Replication Program, a research project sponsored by the National Institute of Justice, showed that children were present in households where domestic violence occurred at *more than twice the rate* at which they were present in comparable households in the general population.

Definitions of what constitutes children's exposure to domestic violence differ, as do research methodologies in this area; estimates of prevalence thus vary widely (Edleson, 1999; Fantuzzo & Mohr, 1999; Osofsky, 2003). In spite of challenging conceptual and methodological issues, research findings to date provide consistent evidence that domestic violence occurs in large numbers of households with children and that domestic violence and child maltreatment are often linked (Fantuzzo & Mohr; Osofsky). The most commonly cited childhood exposure to domestic violence incidence estimates are 3.3 million from the 1975 Family Violence Survey and 10 million from the 1985 Family Violence Survey; these two numbers are frequently combined and cited as a current finding (Carlson, 1984; Straus & Gelles, 1990). In 1998, Holden generated an estimate of 17.8 million children exposed to violence based on Silvern's 1995 study of undergraduates (Holden, 1998; Silvern et al., 1995). Moreover, children who live in homes where domestic violence occurs face an increased risk of child maltreatment. Research studies reveal a 30 to 60% overlap between child abuse/neglect and domestic violence in such families, with a 40% median co-occurrence in the families studied (Edleson, 1999; Edleson, Mbilinyi, Beeman, & Hagemeister, 2003; National Clearinghouse on Child Abuse and Neglect Information, 2000). It is partly because of this overlap that data from the two categories cannot be extrapolated to generate a comprehensive account of the nature and extent of CEV.

Community Violence: Incidence and Prevalence

In neighborhoods nationwide, children and adolescents are victims of homicide, victims of serious violent crime (e.g., rape, robbery, and assault), participants in physical fights, and witnesses to all of these forms of violence. Although juvenile homicide rates in the United States have declined since the early 1990s, they remain unacceptably high (Wilson, 2000). In 2003, 5570 young people ages 10 to 24 were murdered—an average of 15 each day. Juveniles and young adults are also far more likely to be victims of nonfatal violent crime (i.e., rape/sexual assault, robbery, aggravated assault, or simple assault) than persons from other age groups. In 2005, persons age 12 to 15 experienced violent crime at a rate of 44 victimizations per 1000 persons, and persons age 16 to 19 were victimized at a rate of 44.2 per 1000. In comparison, the overall violent crime rate in the United States in 2005 was 21.2 victimizations per 1000 persons age 12 or older (Bureau of Justice Statistics, 2005). In 2004, more than 750,000 young people ages 10 to 24 were treated in emergency departments for injuries sustained due to violence (CDC, 2006c). In a nationwide survey of high school students, 33% reported being in a physical fight one or more times in the 12 months preceding the survey and 17% reported carrying a weapon (e.g., gun, knife, or club) on one or more of the 30 days preceding the survey (CDC, 2006b).

In a review of 43 articles providing quantitative data regarding community violence exposure and three articles reviewing the prevalence of child and adolescent exposure to community violence, Stein, Jaycox, Kataoka, Rhodes, and Vestal (2003) found that prevalence estimates of physical and crime-related community violence exposure range widely, with victimization rates generally lower than witnessing rates. For example, Gladstein, Rusonis, and Heald (1992) reported that 1% of upper middle class youth witnessed a murder, compared to 23% of low-income, predominantly African-American youth, while Fitzpatrick and Boldizar (1993) found that 43% of their predominantly African-American, low-income school-aged child sample reported having witnessed a murder. The percentage of youth who reported witnessing a stabbing in their lifetime ranged from 9% of upper middle class youth (Gladstein et al., 1992) to 56% in a sample of inner city youth (Fitzpatrick & Boldizar, 1993).

School Violence: Incidence and Prevalence

In the 2004–2005 school year, an estimated 54.7 million students were enrolled in pre-kindergarten through grade 12 (National Center for Education Statistics, 2006). While students are less likely to be victims of a violent crime at school than away from school (Dinkes, Cataldi, Kena, & Baum, 2006), exposure to crime and violence at school affects children both directly and indirectly involved and may also disrupt the educational process (Henry, 2000). This is not to imply that violence at school is not a significant source of exposure for children. The percentage of public schools experiencing one or more violent incidents increased between the 1999–2000 and 2003–2004 school years, from 71% to 81% (Dinkes et al., 2006). In 2004, students ages 12–18 were victims of about 1.4 million nonfatal crimes at school, including about 863,000 thefts and 583,000 violent crimes (simple assault and serious violent crime), 107,000 of which were serious violent crimes (rape, sexual assault, robbery, and aggravated assault). These figures represent victimization rates of 33 thefts and 22 violent crimes, including 4 serious violent crimes, per 1000 students at school in 2004 (Dinkes et al., 2006). The total percentage of students who reported the presence of gangs at school increased from 21% in 2003 to 24% in 2005. Students in urban schools were more likely to report the presence of gangs at their school (36%) than students at suburban schools (21%) or rural schools (16%; Dinkes et al., 2006). The presence of gangs more than doubles the likelihood of violent victimization at school (Howell, 2006).

Bullying, in particular, represents a significant source of violence exposure at school (see Song & Stoiber, this issue). In 2005, 28% of students ages 12–18 reported having been bullied at school during the last 6 months (Dinkes et al., 2006). Of these, 58% said that the bullying had happened once or twice during that period, 25% had experienced bullying once or twice a month, 11% reported having been bullied once or twice a week, and 8% said they had been bullied almost daily. Of those students who reported bullying incidents that involved being pushed, shoved, tripped, or spit on (9%), 24% reported that they had sustained an injury ranging in severity from bruising to broken bones to being knocked unconscious during the previous 6 months as a result (Dinkes et al., 2006).

WHY DON'T WE KNOW MORE? CHALLENGES TO MEASURING THE NATURE AND EXTENT OF CEV

As recognition about the co-occurrence of types of exposure, as well as the chronicity of exposure grows, as children cross multiple service paths, and as the profound impact of exposure on child development continues to be documented, there is an ongoing shift in the field toward a broader conceptualization of CEV. Unfortunately, researchers and practitioners face a number of significant challenges in their efforts to develop a comprehensive picture of CEV that is supported by robust data on incidence and prevalence. These challenges have been identified in a series of professional meetings, including the 2002 Workshop on Children Exposed to Violence: Current Status, Gaps, and Research Priorities (Analytical Sciences, Inc., 2002) and the *Think Tank on Children Exposed to Violence* (Institute on Violence, Abuse, and Trauma, 2006). They have also been explored in a number of publications (Finkelhor et al., 2005; Geffner, Jaffe, & Sudermann, 2000; Graham-Berman & Edleson, 2001; Guterman, 2004; Jaffe, Baker, & Cunningham, 2004), most recently in *Children Exposed to Violence* (Feerick & Silverman, 2006). The following sections are intended to introduce the practitioner to the key issues related to collecting, analyzing, and interpreting data that supports a comprehensive picture of CEV.

Definitions

Researchers and practitioners lack a common language in which to conduct and discuss research, prevention, and intervention related to CEV. Key terms such as *exposure* and *violence* are used inconsistently within CEV literature, and sometimes even within the same article. For example, *exposure* is used to describe the child's involvement or experience in multiple ways, referring at times to a child who witnesses but does not experience abuse directly and at other times to direct victimization. The term exposure is also used to characterize an event during which a child was exposed, and to attribute psychological impact to an event. The term "exposure" has been used to encompass varying levels of traumatic occurrences, ranging from single, acute acts to repeated or chronic events.

It is difficult to precisely define exposure in part because we lack a precise definition of violence. While it is useful to begin by defining *violence* as an act of harm or intent to harm, *exposure* needs to be concretely conceptualized in terms of type, severity, frequency, timing, proximity, and relationship to victim or perpetrator in order to provide a firm and consistent foundation for investigation. The lack of this firm foundation has been widely acknowledged, identified as a barrier to research (Runyan et al., 2005), and addressed to some extent particularly within domestic violence and child abuse literature (Holden, 2003). Research is an appropriate means for developing CEV definitions. At the same time, research progress is predicated on having standard definitions, since without nationally standardized and accepted definitions for various forms of violence, researchers must independently determine categorizations and definitions for the purposes of their research. These independently developed definitions can be both appropriate and methodologically sound, but their variation contributes to research findings that are not easily compared.

Fragmentation

Historically, the environmental context in which violence occurred, the nature/type of violence, or the service pathway through which the child's exposure became known has been used to define the exposure. Researchers and practitioners have worked almost exclusively in "silos" defined by the type of violence exposure. The still-emerging field of CEV has previously been numerous different fields, which have been discretely defined and have evolved and matured independently, tackling research and service agendas without a comparative or integrative perspective (Miller-Perrin, 2006). This fragmentation within the field has far-reaching effects. First, current CEV estimates, which are based on data gathered within but not across the discrete fields, are likely to underrepresent the magnitude of the problem (Finkelhor et al., 2005). Data gathered in this way also fail to highlight the interrelationships of CEV (Finkelhor et al., 2005; Lynch, 2006). Interrelationships include the co-occurrence of types of violence (e.g., domestic violence and child maltreatment), associations such as multiple incidents of the same type of event (such as bullying), and the heightened vulnerability of some child victims for further and different types of victimizations (Finkelhor et al., 2005).

Dynamic Nature of the Problem

From a measurement perspective, it is important to understand that a variety of factors contribute to a child's position on what Betsy McAlister-Groves, founding director of the Child Witness to Violence Project at Boston Medical Center, has termed the "stress to trauma continuum." Children exhibit a wide range of responses to adversity. The effects of violence vary greatly from child to child, and are influenced by factors that contribute to these effects, including proximity to the event, severity of the event, the child's gender and age, the chronicity of exposure, the child's relationship to the victim and perpetrator, and the presence of other stressors (Garmezy, 1993; Jenkins & Bell, 1994; Nader, Pynoos, Fairbanks, & Frederick, 1990; Singer, Anglin, Song, & Lunghofer, 1995).

Not all children exposed to violence exhibit signs of maladjustment or adverse impacts. Moreover, some children may show resilience, which is defined as not simply the absence of pathology but the presence of competence in the face of crisis (Kitzmann, Gaylord, Holt, & Kenny, 2003). Protective factors such as family situation, community environment, and the existence of a positive and supportive relationship between the child and a caring adult can help foster resilience (Luthar, 2006). Factors related to risk and resilience have been summarized into three groups: factors related to the child, characteristics of the event, and characteristics of the family and social system (Perry & Azad, 1999). These individual factors must be taken into consideration both when designing methodology and drawing conclusions from aggregate data regarding particular events, in that each event may create a vastly different experience for any individual child. Furthermore, such variations contribute to difficulties in understanding dose/response relationships between exposure and pathology in children exposed to violence.

While neuroscientists are now documenting and labeling traumatic events, experiences, and ongoing adversity as *toxic stress*, the level and degree that constitutes toxicity has not been determined (National Scientific Council on the Developing Child, 2005). Discussions at the Institute on Violence, Abuse, and Trauma's (2006) *Think Tank on Children Exposed to Violence* centered in part on this complexity and gap in knowledge. The stress-to-trauma continuum acknowledges that all events are not traumatic and that stress over time can have at least as great an impact on children as a single traumatic event. This concept of stress moving toward toxic levels on a continuum captures the dynamic nature of the problem.

Other Challenges

The development of research designs and methodologies capable of capturing the range of children's experiences within a developmental framework and considering the implications of gender, culture, ethnicity, political context, and child disability along with the development of new theoretical models that expand understanding about the effects of CEV are two areas where significant work remains to be done (Feerick & Silverman, 2006). In addition to methodological challenges, the process of obtaining comprehensive data on the extent and nature of CEV is hampered by myths and misconceptions about violence, as well as societal variations as to what constitutes violence. Moreover, silence about the problem leads to underreporting of all types of violence, particularly violence in the home.

FACING THE CHALLENGES: WHERE DO WE GO FROM HERE?

Within the last 15 to 20 years, research literature has emerged in recognition of the impact of CEV beyond direct victimization (Edleson, 2004). There is general agreement among researchers and practitioners that an ecological and transactional model is needed to fully understand the complexity of CEV and address the problem (Dawes & Donald, 2000; Kracke & Cohen, 2008, this issue). Childen exposed to violence must be understood in the context of the interrelationships of the child to the family, caregivers, and community in the face of a violent event, as well as in the context of the developmental stage in which the event occurred and any previous events (Dawes & Donald, 2000). It is essential that research begin to comprehensively capture the nature and extent of CEV, which is inherently both complex and dynamic even in response to single events. Only then can we begin to extricate and address the many factors that influence a child's response to violence and begin to craft targeted and effective interventions.

As understanding of the impact of CEV has grown, perceptions and categorizations of children's exposure have also broadened. This expanded view is significant in its potential to improve the way children and their families are served in all social service systems, not only by improving the effectiveness of the interventions and supports, but also by realigning systems around the family's strengths and needs in an ecological context. Such a holistic view of violence in the context of a child and his/her family can serve to break down silos across disciplines that have developed independently for decades.

To accomplish this, practitioners, policymakers, and researchers first need to agree upon a joint agenda that can inform both policy and practice. Such an agenda might begin with the further development and implementation of a common and consistent vocabulary for describing CEV. A common language provides the foundation for further research, reducing barriers to collecting and comparing data and bringing consistency in research methodology as well as in approach to collaborative efforts at the direct practice and policy levels.

In 1999, CDC published *Version 1.0* of *Intimate Partner Violence Surveillance: Uniform Definitions and Recommended Data Elements* (Saltzman, Fanslow, McMahon, & Shelley, 1999). In 2002, CDC published *Version 1.0* of *Sexual Violence Surveillance: Uniform Definitions and Recommended Data Elements* (Basile, & Saltzman, 2002). Currently, a third document in this series of *Uniform Definitions and Recommended Data Elements* is being drafted, which will define child maltreatment and associated terms based on the consensus of professionals in child maltreatment research (Leeb, Paulozzi, Melanson, Simon, & Arias, 2006). These documents represent excellent progress toward the goal of developing common language in these individual violence subtypes, but these documents need to be expanded if we are to adopt a larger perspective on the impact of violence on children. If developed as a companion to the series, a fourth document could provide uniform definitions and recommended data elements on children's exposure to violence. This document would then also lay the groundwork needed for the development of a public surveillance system that acknowledges and addresses CEV as a critical public health problem.

Second, the development and implementation of methodologies that look across the traditionally independent fields of CEV as defined by exposure type, as well as address the measurement of chronicity, severity, and co-occurrence of types of violence, is required in order to adequately capture the magnitude of the problem. In response, the U.S. Department of Justice (DOJ) under the Office of Juvenile Justice and Delinquency Prevention (OJJDP) is funding and coordinating a National Survey of Children's Exposure to Violence (NATSCEV). Conducted by Drs. David Finkelhor, Heather Turner, and associates at the University of New Hampshire, this study will utilize and expand upon the DVS as the most extensive survey data currently available. The NATSCEV will enhance the DVS' JVQ to collect more comprehensive CEV incidence and prevalence data. Currently in the design phase and with survey implementation scheduled to commence by 2008, this study proposes to use telephone survey methodology to obtain a target sample of 4000–6000 children ages 2–17 (Finkelhor, Turner, Hamby, & Holt, 2007). The assessment will incorporate a broad range of victimization experiences across a wide developmental spectrum to examine a variety of potential predictors and outcomes of CEV as discussed and recommended throughout this article. In collaboration between OJJDP and CDC, the study will also collect outcomes on safe, stable, and nurturing relationships, which will provide additional information on protective influences in children's lives.

Third, a public surveillance system on children's exposure to violence needs to be established, as called for by practitioners and researchers who recognize the breadth of the problem as a public health concern (Fantuzzo, Mohr, & Noone, 2000). Through a national surveillance system, the network of disciplines, policymakers, practitioners, and researchers can begin to know the full extent of violence in children's lives; share responsibility for addressing the problem; and measure progress towards effectively preventing and reducing the impacts of this exposure to violence over time.

Finally, further examination of the extent and degree of CEV and its characteristics should inform the development of a more comprehensive and reliable package of screening and assessment tools for a full range of practitioners (including nonclinical service providers) at all points along the continuum (prevention, intervention, treatment, and response). Equipped with such enhanced assessment tools, mental health providers and CEV professionals will be better able to assess the psychosocial health of children across developmental stages. In particular, work needs to be done in the development of screening and assessment tools for young children (Stover & Berkowitz, 2005).

THE IMPORTANCE OF MEETING THE CHALLENGES

Even without specific numbers to document the nature and extent of CEV, the welfare of children exposed to violence has become a major concern as continued research demonstrates the harmful effects of exposure (Edmond, Fitzgerald, & Kracke, 2005). In brief, this research continues to indicate the devastating impact of child maltreatment (Widom, 2000), family violence (Edleson, 1999; Osofsky 1999), community violence (Brill, Fiorentino, & Grant, 2001; Lynch, 2003; Lynch & Cicchetti 1998), and school violence (Henry, 2000) on vulnerable children and on society in general. The impact of exposure extends to neurological development, physical health, mental health, school performance, substance use/abuse, and risk behaviors. The impact data provides some indications of the relative risks of different populations, and indicates that even very young children are adversely affected by exposure to violence, with children aged 2 years and younger exhibiting symptoms such as sleep disturbances, flashbacks, separation anxiety, aggression, hyperactivity, and emotional detachment (Carlson, 2000; Graham-Bermann, 2002; Perry, 1997; Pynoos & Nader, 1986; Shonkoff & Phillips, 2000; Terr, 1991).

Documentation of the impact of exposure is coupled with a growing awareness that children exposed to violence often do not receive adequate intervention or treatment to address harmful after effects (Edmond et al., 2005). Researchers and practitioners are beginning to learn more about prevention and intervention measures and strategies. The literature reflects limited but growing efforts to document intervention practices and to demonstrate efficacy in intervention strategies, and resource allocation and public investment in the issue have grown at federal, state, and local levels in the last 10 years.

This is excellent progress, but we must do more. Comprehensive data documenting the incidence and prevalence of CEV at both the local and national level is essential to the efforts of researchers, practitioners, and policymakers to realistically assess the scope of the problem and meaningfully address it in proportion to its magnitude. Gaps in such data exist both nationally and locally, limiting the abilities of practitioners and policymakers to define the scope of the problem and to collaboratively plan for more comprehensive and responsive service delivery systems to prevent and reduce the impacts of CEV (Association for the Study and Development of Community [ASDC], 2007). Efforts to capture local prevalence through the Safe Start initiative (supported by OJJDP and described in Kracke and Cohen (2008, this issue) have been challenged by a lack of available data and consistent measurement. Prevalence estimates captured through case analysis and rough data, however, further suggest that the scope of the problem is much greater than currently documented, even after factoring in accepted general challenges related to underreporting and societal/cultural variations about violence, relationships, families, and privacy (ASDC, 2007; Shields, 2006). Each attempt, nationally and locally, to collect robust numbers has increased estimates regarding the real extent of the problem.

Enhanced data on the nature and extent of CEV can be used to increase awareness about the potential harm to our children and challenges societal attitudes toward violence. Social marketing and public education strategies for both practitioners and the general public were shown to be both critical and effective in changing systems to better respond to children exposed to violence in the Safe Start demonstration sites (ASDC, 2007; Kracke & Cohen, 2008, this issue). A full description of the Safe Start demonstration sites and the evaluation findings can be found in *The Safe Start Initiative: Building and Disseminating Knowledge to Support Children Exposed to Violence* (see Kracke & Cohen, 2008, this issue).

Robust and comprehensive data increases awareness in the field itself and provides documented evidence of the need for more resources, science, and cross-disciplinary service integration as well as better practice tools to transform a service delivery system to more appropriately and effectively address the needs of families. An appropriate understanding of the problem helps drive the allocation of resources to develop more evidence-based practice. Once we more fully understand the aggregate problem, we can more effectively dissect and disentangle the other factors influencing risk and resiliency, acuteness and chronicity, and stress and trauma. A mindful understanding of the problem challenges us to broaden our perspectives and define exposure more inclusively and ecologically. Only then can we understand and effectively respond to support children and their families living in violence and adversity, thereby disrupting the stress to trauma continuum and re-establishing an environment for healthy development.

REFERENCES

Analytical Sciences, Inc. (2002). *Children exposed to violence: Current status, gaps, and research priorities.* Workshop Summary of the NICHD Workshop on Children Exposed to Violence, Washington, DC.

Association for the Study and Development of Community (ASDC). (2007). *Creating comprehensive and responsive systems of care for children exposed to violence: The Safe Start demonstration project: Process evaluation report 2000–2005.* Gaithersburg, MD: Author.

Basile, K. C., & Saltzman L. E. (2002). *Sexual violence surveillance: Uniform definitions and recommended data elements.* Atlanta, GA: Centers for Disease Control and Prevention, National Center for Injury Prevention and Control.

Brill, C., Fiorentino, N., & Grant, J. (2001). Covictimization and inner city youth: A review. *International Journal of Emergency Mental Health, 3*(4), 229–239.

Bureau of Justice Statistics. (2005). *A National Crime Victimization Survey, 2005 - Statistical tables NCJ 215244.* Washington, DC: U.S. Department of Justice, Office of Justice Programs. Retrieved April 20, 2007, from http://www.ojp.usdoj.gov/bjs/

Carlson, B. E. (1984). Children's observations of interpersonal violence. In A. Roberts (Ed.), *Battered men and their families* (pp. 147–167). New York: Springer.

Carlson, B. E. (2000). Children exposed to intimate partner violence: Research findings and implications for intervention. *Trauma, Violence, & Abuse, 1,* 321–342.

Catalano, S. (2006). *Intimate partner violence in the United States.* Special Report. Washington, DC: U.S. Department of Justice, Office of Justice Programs, Bureau of Justice Statistics. Retrieved February 13, 2007, from http://www.ojp.usdoj.gov/bjs/intimate/ipv.htm

Centers for Disease Control and Prevention. (2003). *Costs of intimate partner violence against women in the United States.* Atlanta, GA: National Center for Injury Prevention and Control. Retrieved September 13, 2007, from http://www.cdc.gov/ncipc/pub-res/ipv_cost/IPVBook-Final-Feb18.pdf

Centers for Disease Control and Prevention. (2006a). *Major findings.* Atlanta, GA: U.S. Department of Health and Human Services. Retrieved September 16, 2007, from http://www.cdc.gov/nccdphp/ace/findings.htm

Centers for Disease Control and Prevention. (2006b). *2005 youth risk behavior survey*. Atlanta, GA: U.S. Department of Health and Human Services. Retrieved April 20, 2007, from www.cdc.gov/yrbss

Centers for Disease Control and Prevention. (2006c). *Web-based injury statistics query and reporting system (WISQARS)*. National Center for Injury Prevention and Control. Atlanta, GA: U.S. Department of Health and Human Services. Retrieved April 27, 2007, from http://www.cdc.gov/ncipc/wisqars

Children's Bureau. (2005a). *Child maltreatment 2005*. Washington, DC: U.S. Department of Health and Human Services, Administration for Children and Families, Administration on Children, Youth, and Families.

Children's Bureau. (2005b). National Incidence Study of Child Abuse and Neglect. *Children's Bureau Express*, July/August 2005, 6(6). Washington, DC: U.S. Department of Health and Human Services, Administration for Children and Families, Administration on Children, Youth, and Families. Retrieved September 7, 2007, from http://cbexpress.acf.hhs.gov

Dawes, A., & Donald, D. (2000). Improving children's chances: Developmental theory and effective interventions in community contexts. In D. Donald, A. Dawes, & J. Louw (Eds.), *Addressing childhood adversity* (pp. 1–25.). Cape Town, South Africa: David Philip.

Dilillo, D., Tremblay, G., & Peterson, L. (2000). Maternal anger. *Child Abuse and Neglect, 24*(6), 767–779.

Dinkes, R., Cataldi, E. F., Kena, G., & Baum, K. (2006). *Indicators of school crime and safety: 2006*. Washington, DC: U.S. Department of Education, National Center for Education Statistics; & U.S. Department of Justice, Office of Justice Programs, Bureau of Justice Statistics. Retrieved April 20, 2007, from http://nces.ed.gov/programs/crimeindicators/

Edleson, J. L. (1999). Children's witnessing of adult domestic violence. *Journal of Interpersonal Violence, 14*(8), 839–870.

Edleson, J. L. (2004). Should childhood exposure to adult domestic violence be defined as child maltreatment under the law? In P. Jaffe, L. Baker, & A. Cunningham (Eds.), *Protecting children from domestic violence: Strategies for community intervention* (pp. 8–29). New York: Guilford Press.

Edleson, J. L., Mbilinyi, L. F., Beeman, S. K., & Hagemeister, A. K. (2003). How children are involved in adult domestic violence: Results from a four-city telephone survey. *Journal of Interpersonal Violence, 18*(1), 18–32.

Edmond, Y., Fitzgerald, M., & Kracke, K. (2005). *Incidence and prevalence of CEV 2005*. Washington, DC: Author. Retrieved September 14, 2007, from http://www.safestartcenter.org

Fantuzzo, J. W., & Mohr, W. K. (1999). Prevalence and effects of child exposure to domestic violence. *The Future of Children, 9*(3), 21–32. Retrieved December 22, 2003, from http://www.futureofchildren.org

Fantuzzo, J. W., Mohr, W. K., & Noone, M. J. (2000). Making the invisible victims of violence against women visible through university/community partnerships. In R. Geffner, P. Jaffe, & M. Sudermann (Eds.) *Children exposed to domestic violence: Current issues in research, intervention, prevention, and policy development* (pp. 9–23). Binghamton, NY: Haworth Press.

Feerick, M., & Silverman, G. (Eds.). (2006). *Children exposed to violence*. Baltimore, MD: Paul H. Brookes Publishing.

Felitti, V. J., Anda, R. F., Nordenberg, D., Williamson, D. F., Spitz, A. M., Edwards, V., et al. (1998). Relationship of childhood abuse and household dysfunction to many of the leading causes of death in adults: The Adverse Childhood Experiences (ACE) Study. *American Journal of Preventive Medicine, 14*(4), 245–258.

Finkelhor, D., Ormrod, R., Turner, H., & Hamby, S. L. (2005). The victimization of children and youth: A comprehensive, national survey. *Child Maltreatment, 10*, 5–25.

Finkelhor, D., Turner, H., Hamby, S., & Holt, M. (2007). *National survey of children's exposure to violence: Progress report to the U.S. Department of Justice's Office of Juvenile Justice and Delinquency Prevention*. Unpublished manuscript.

Fitzpatrick, K. M., & Boldizar, J. P. (1993). The prevalence and consequences of exposure to violence among African-American youth. *Journal of the American Academy of Child and Adolescent Psychiatry, 32*, 424–430.

Frierson, T. A. (1999). The prevalence and impact of exposure to violence among emotionally disturbed/behaviorally disordered boys. Unpublished doctoral dissertation. *Dissertation Abstracts International, 60*(7–A), 2444.

Garmezy, N. (1993). Children in poverty: Resilience despite risk. *Psychiatry: Interpersonal and Biological Processes, 56*, 127–136.

Geffner, R. A., Jaffe, P. G., & Sudermann, M. (Eds.). (2000). *Children exposed to domestic violence: Current issues in research, intervention, prevention, and policy development*. Binghamton, NY: Haworth Press.

Gladstein, J., Rusonis, E. J., & Heald, F. P. (1992). A comparison of inner-city and upper middle class youth's exposure to violence. *Journal of Adolescent Health, 13*, 275–280.

Graham-Bermann, S. A. (2002). Child abuse in the context of domestic violence. In J. E. B. Myers & L. Berliner (Eds.), *The APSAC handbook on child maltreatment* (2nd ed., pp. 119–129). Thousand Oaks, CA: Sage Publications.

Graham-Bermann, S. A., & Edleson, J. L. (Eds.). (2001). *Domestic violence in the lives of children: The future of research, intervention, and social policy*. Washington, DC: American Psychological Association.

Guterman, N. B. (2004). Advancing prevention research on child abuse, youth violence, and domestic violence: Emerging strategies and issues. *Journal of Interpersonal Violence, 19*(3), 299–321.

Henry, S. (2000). What is school violence? An integrated definition. *Annals of the American Academy of Political and Social Science, 567*, 16–29.

Holden, G. W. (1998). Introduction: The development of research into another consequence of family violence. In G. W. Holden, R. Geffner, & E. N. Jouriles (Eds.), *Children exposed to marital violence: Theory, research, and applied issues* (pp. 1–18). Washington, DC: American Psychological Association.

Holden, G. W. (2003). Children exposed to domestic violence and child abuse: Terminology and taxonomy. *Clinical Child and Family Psychology Review, 6*(3), 151–160.

Howell, J. C. (2006). *The impact of gangs on communities*. Washington, DC: U.S. Department of Justice, Office of Juvenile Justice and Delinquency Prevention, NYGC Bulletin. Retrieved April 20, 2007, from http://www.iir.com/nygc/

Institute on Violence, Abuse, and Trauma. (2006). Meeting minutes from the Children Exposed to Violence National *Think Tank*. 11th International Conference on Violence, Abuse, and Trauma, September 14–19, San Diego, CA.

Jaffe, P. G., Baker, L. L., & Cunningham, A. J. (2004). *Protecting children from domestic violence: Strategies from domestic violence: Strategies for community intervention*. New York: Guilford Press.

Jenkins, E. J., & Bell, C. C. (1994). Violence exposure, psychological distress, and high risk behaviors in a sample of inner-city youth. In S. Friedman (Ed.), *Anxiety disorders in African-Americans* (pp. 76–88) New York: Springer.

Kitzmann, K. M., Gaylord, N. K., Holt, A. R., & Kenny, E. D. (2003). Child witnesses to domestic violence: A meta-analytic review. *Journal of Consulting and Clinical Psychology, 71*(2), 339–352.

Kracke, K., & Cohen, E. (2008). The Safe Start Initiative: Building and disseminating knowledge to support children exposed to violence. *Journal of Emotional Abuse, 8*(1/2), 155–174.

Leeb, R. T., Paulozzi, L., Melanson C., Simon, T., & Arias I. (2006). *Child maltreatment surveillance: Uniform definitions for public health and recommended data elements, Version 1.0.* Atlanta, GA: Centers for Disease Control and Prevention, National Center for Injury Prevention and Control.

Luthar, S. S. (2006). Resilience in development: A synthesis of research across five decades. In D. Cicchetti & D. J. Cohen (Eds.), *Developmental psychopathology: Risk, disorder, and adaptation* (2nd ed., pp. 740–795). New York: John Wiley & Sons.

Lynch, M. (2003). Consequences of children's exposure to community violence. *Clinical Child and Family Psychology Review, 6*, 265–274.

Lynch, M. (2006). Children exposed to community violence. In M. M. Feerick & G. B. Silverman (Eds.), *Children exposed to violence* (pp. 29–52). Baltimore, MD: Paul H. Brookes Publishing.

Lynch, M., & Cicchetti, D. (1998). An ecological-transactional analysis of children and contexts: The longitudinal interplay among child maltreatment, community violence and children's symptomatology. *Development and Psychopathology, 10*, 235–257.

Miller-Perrin, C. (2006). Growing up in a violent world: It's not child's play. *PsycCRITIQUES, 51*(28).

Nader, K., Pynoos, R. S., Fairbanks, L., & Frederick, C. (1990). Childhood PTSD reactions one year after sniper attack. *Journal of the American Psychiatric Association, 147*, 1526–1530.

National Center for Education Statistics. (2006). *Digest of education statistics, 2005*. Washington, DC: U.S. Department of Education. Retrieved from April 22, 2007, from http://nces.ed.gov/programs/digest/d05/index.asp

National Clearinghouse on Child Abuse and Neglect Information. (2000). *In harm's way: Domestic violence and child maltreatment*. Washington, DC: U.S. Government Printing Office.

National Scientific Council on the Developing Child. (2005). *Excessive stress disrupts the architecture of the developing brain* (Working Paper No. 3). Retrieved February 12, 2007, from http://www.developingchild.net/pubs/wp/excessive stress.pdf

Osofsky, J. D. (1999). The impact of violence on children. *Future of Children, 9*, 33–49.

Osofsky, J. D. (2003). Prevalence of children's exposure to domestic violence and child maltreatment: Implications for prevention and intervention. *Clinical Child and Family Psychology Review, 6*(3), 161–170.

Perry, B. D. (1997). Incubated in terror: Neurodevelopmental factors in the "cycle of violence." In J. D. Osofsky (Ed.), *Children, youth, and violence: The search for solutions* (pp. 124–148). New York: Guilford Press.

Perry, B. D., & Azad, I. (1999). Post-traumatic stress disorders in children and adolescents. *Current Opinions in Pediatrics, 11*(4), 121–132.

Pynoos, R. S., & Nader, K. (1986). Children's exposure to violence and traumatic death. *Psychiatric Annals, 20*, 334–344.

Rennison, C. M., & Rand, M. R. (2003). *Criminal victimization, 2002.* Washington, DC: U.S. Department of Justice, Office of Justice Programs, Bureau of Justice Statistics. Retrieved January 9, 2007, from http://www.ojp.usdoj.gov/bjs

Runyan, D. K, Cox, C. E., Dubowitz, H., Newton, R. R., Upadhyaya, M., Kotch, J. B, et al. (2005). Describing maltreatment: Do child protective service reports and research definitions agree? *Child Abuse & Neglect, 29*(5), 461–477.

Saltzman L. E., Fanslow J. L., McMahon P. M., & Shelley G. A. (1999). *Intimate partner violence surveillance: Uniform definitions and recommended data elements, Version 1.0.* Atlanta, GA: Centers for Disease Control and Prevention, National Center for Injury Prevention and Control.

Sedlak, A. J., & Broadhurst, D. D. (1996). *Executive summary of the Third National Incidence Study of Child Abuse and Neglect.* Washington, DC: U.S. Department of Health and Human Services, Administration for Children and Families, Administration on Children, Youth and Families, National Center of Child Abuse and Neglect. Retrieved September 7, 2007, from http://www.childwelfare.gov/pubs/statsinfo/nis3.cfm

Shields, J. P. (2006). *I tried to stop them: Children's exposure to domestic violence in San Francisco.* San Francisco, CA: Education, Training, & Research Associates.

Shonkoff, J. P., & Phillips, D. A. (2000). *From neurons to neighborhoods: The science of early childhood development.* Washington, DC: National Academy Press.

Silvern, L., Karyl, J., Waelde, L., Hodges, W.F., Starek, J., Heidt, E., et al. (1995). Retrospective reports of parental partner abuse: Relationships to depression, trauma symptoms and self-esteem among college students. *Journal of Family Violence, 10*, 177–201.

Singer, M. I., Anglin, T. M., Song, L. Y., & Lunghofer, L. (1995). Adolescents' exposure to violence and associated symptoms of psychological trauma. *Journal of the American Medical Association, 273*, 477–482.

Song, S. Y., & Stoiber, K. (2008). Children exposed to violence at school: An evidence-based intervention agenda for the "real" bullying problem. *Journal of Emotional Abuse, 8*(1/2), 235–253.

Stein B. D., Jaycox, L. H., Kataoka, S., Rhodes, H. J., & Vestal, K. D. (2003). Prevalence of child and adolescent exposure to community violence. *Clinical Child and Family Psychology Review, 6*(4), 247–264.

Stover, C., & Berkowitz, S. J. (2005). A critical review of PTSD measures for young children. *The International Journal of Traumatic Stress, 18*(6), 707–717.

Straus, M. A. (1991, September). *Children as witness to material violence: A risk factor for life long problems among a nationally representative sample of American men and women*. Paper presented at the Ross Round Table Children and Violence, Washington, DC.

Straus, M. A., & Gelles, R. J. (1990). *Physical violence in American families*. New Brunswick, NJ: Transaction.

Terr, L. (1991). Childhood traumas: An outline and an overview. *American Journal of Psychiatry, 48*, 10–20.

Widom, C. S. (2000). Understanding the consequences of childhood victimization. In R. M. Reece (Ed.), *Treatment of child abuse* (pp. 339–361). Baltimore, MD: Johns Hopkins University Press.

Wilson, J. J. (2000). *Children as victims*. Bulletin. Washington, DC: U.S. Department of Justice, Office of Justice Programs, Office of Juvenile Justice and Delinquency Prevention. Retrieved January 9, 2004, from http://www.ojjdp.ncjrs.org

Violence and the Effects of Trauma on American Indian and Alaska Native Populations

Sadie Willmon-Haque
Dolores Subia BigFoot

It is impossible to capture and adequately explain the complex nature and extent of devastation experienced by American Indian/Alaska Native[1] (AI/AN) families since the "discovery of the New World" (BigFoot & Braden, 2007; Weaver, 1998). From the 1490's to the 1890's, "Europeans and white Americans engaged in an unbroken string of genocide campaigns against the Native people of the Americas" (Stannard, 1992,

p. 147). The political, social, and economic policies of the 20th Century did not offer much change. Instead, several generations of AI/AN were the recipients of violent assaults resulting in high levels of traumatic exposure (also see Chamberlain, 2008, this issue, for a discussion on historical trauma and cultural issues).

Trauma and violence among AI/AN populations are significant and emerging topics in scientific and community-based literature. Several meaningful books and peer-reviewed articles have been recently published on their exposure to trauma due to colonialization, racism, out-of-home placements, substance abuse, and other destructive behaviors (e.g., Deters, Novins, Fickenscher, & Beals, 2006; Duran, 2006; Ehlers et al., 2006; Evans-Campbell, Lindhorst, Huang, & Walters, 2006; Harwell, Moore, & Spence, 2003; Kaufman, Beals, Mitchell, LeMaster, & Fickenscher, 2004; Strickland, Walsh, & Cooper, 2006). Other outlets such as national centers, professional associations, and agencies have focused on the connection between trauma, violence, and mental and physical health among AI/AN, including the Indian Country Child Trauma Center (www.icctc.org); American Indian and Alaska Native Summit on Suicide Prevention, Intervention, and Healing (www.nicwa.org); Indian Health Service (IHS) Director's Initiatives (www.ihs.gov); and Association of American Indian Physicians (www.aaip.org).

Vulnerability to trauma is related to the damaging social conditions and multiple marginalization facing AI/AN people (BigFoot, 2000; McCabe, 2007). Vulnerability to trauma was created under conditions of poverty, historical trauma, and cultural hegemony adding susceptibility for the layers of violence now well established in tribal communities.

DIVERSITY OF CULTURES AND SHARED BELIEFS AMONG INDIGENOUS PEOPLE

Historically and culturally, the indigenous people of the New World consisted of numerous separate and diverse groups, some connected by alliances or language but each having their own beliefs, customs, rituals, ceremonies, and territories. Most possessed creation stories that spoke of their origin and their way of life. Within their stories, passed from generation to generation, they were taught how to treat each other, their relationships to the land and the other creations (animals, earth, and sky), their sources for food, shelter, guidance, and good favor, and the purpose of their journey in this world. They knew about and were respectful of the seasons, which brought either blessings or demise. They also knew and were respectful of the elements; for example, if one disrespected water then one could drown or be pulled under by the spirits who lived below the water. Finally, they knew and were respectful of the forces of nature; for example, if one disrespected the wind, those spirits could carry one away and leave orphans of ones children.

In a recent qualitative study, House, Stiffman, and Brown (2006) found that recognizing oneself as a part of and valuing the community was viewed as important to American Indians and tribal ethnic identity among youth, parents, and elders. Ceremonies, with the underlying goal of offering thanks and maintaining a strong sense of connection through harmony and balance of mind, body, and spirit with the natural environment (Garrett, Garrett, & Brotherton, 2001), are ways that AI/AN have nurtured a sense of belonging among community members.

While it is not possible to give a detailed explanation of the diversity of the tribal groups or the various teachings that exist among groups, certain shared values exist among most groups. These values include cherishing family network and the extended family relationships, beliefs about generosity and sharing, valuing of elders and wisdom, respect for nature and nature's ways, and the interdependency among members. Shared values were necessary for survival since survival was dependent on trust and sharing of resources.[2]

POVERTY AND AI/AN

There were 2.5 million self-identified AI/AN in the 2000 Census, 38% which were under the age of 18, indicating that the AI/AN population is young (Ogunwole, 2002; U.S. Census Bureau, 2000) and in need of care. Nationally, AI/ANs have the highest poverty rates of all racial/ethnic populations (U.S. Census Bureau, 2000; Zuckerman, Haley, Roubideaux, & Lillie-Blanton, 2004). Zuckerman et al. (2004) found from the National Survey of America's Families that 55% of AI/AN have incomes below 200% of the federal poverty level. It has been suggested by Bouman

(2006), Director of Advocacy of the Sargent Shriver National Center on Poverty Law (http://www.povertylaw.org/), that "there seems to be a solid consensus that people who live at 200% of the Federal Poverty Level (FPL) have many of the same problems as those who live below it." It can be suggested from this data that about one in two American Indians struggle to make ends meet. Educational attainment and secure employment are inversely related to poverty. It is thus not surprising that 20% of AI/AN live in families in which no adult graduated from high school (Zuckerman et al., 2004), which makes employability more difficult.

American Indian/Alaska Native women face many financial hardships. Their obligations are often overwhelming because their skill level is not marketable but their familial responsibilities are broad (La Fromboise & Heyle, 1990). For example, AI/AN women retain extended family obligations and responsibilities although doing so often carries a tremendous financial and psychological burden (BigFoot, 1989). For instance, it is not uncommon for AI/AN women to take care of family members with chronic illnesses (e.g., diabetes and substance abuse) or those who have virtually no where else to go but the streets.

In addition, AI/AN elders who are increasingly caring for their grandchildren also face more poverty. In 2000, about half of AI/AN grandparents age 45 and older in the U.S had been raising a grandchild for 5 years or longer (Fuller-Thomson & Minkler, 2005). They found that one-third of grandparent caregivers were living below the poverty line and only one-quarter of them were receiving public assistance. Despite these circumstances, it was found that grandparents were committed to raising their grandchildren though they were disproportionately female, poor, living with a functional disability, and living in overcrowded conditions.

HISTORICAL TRAUMA AND AI/AN TRIBES, FAMILIES, AND INDIVIDUALS

Historical trauma involves exposure of an earlier generation to a traumatic event that continues to affect subsequent generations (Cole, 2006). The effects of historical trauma on the AI/AN family (clans, bands, societies) included colonization by a dominant force that was patriarchal and patrilineal (Cole, 2006). In most cases, misogyny (hatred or prejudice against women) and the impairment of parenting skills were largely due to the removal of adults from their role as caregivers through the boarding school movement (Colmont et al., 2004). Cole indicated that such breakdowns in family relationships can be seen in the high level of child abuse and domestic violence in AI/AN families. For instance, there is approximately one substantiated report of a child victim of abuse or neglect for every 30 AI/AN children (National Child Abuse and Neglect Data System, 2002). In addition, AI/AN children are one of the two most overrepresented groups in child protective services and are represented at twice their proportions in the census populations in the foster care system (Hill, 2006).

The effects of historical trauma on the AI/AN individual may include the development of post-traumatic stress disorder (PTSD; Cole, 2006). Cole emphasized the complexity of the impact of historical trauma on the psychological well-being of AIs:

> The most frequent co-morbid diagnoses with PTSD, outside of other anxiety disorders, include depression and substance abuse. A full evaluation must account for these diagnoses. In the area of substance abuse, the use or abuse of substances can be seen as self-protective. (pp. 124–125)

Although historical trauma has not yet been consistently found to be a precursor to traumatic stress disorders, it creates a pathway in which the members of that culture are at greater risk of experiencing psychological disturbances, becoming less able to draw on the strengths of their culture, family, or natural network for social and emotional support (BigFoot & Braden, 2007).

DEFINING TRAUMA WITH AI/AN POPULATIONS

Trauma symptoms impact a person's emotional, behavioral, cognitive, and psychobiological domains (Cohen, Mannarino, & Deblinger, 2006). According to the National Child Traumatic Stress Network (NCTSN; 2005), trauma is a unique individual experience associated with a traumatic event or enduring conditions that can involve death or other loss, serious injury, or threat to a child's well-being. However, BigFoot and Braden (2007) reported that "this definition is of limited usefulness within AI/AN communities since it does not take into account the cultural trauma, historical trauma, and intergenerational trauma that has accumulated in AI/AN communities through centuries of exposure to racism, warfare, violence, and catastrophic disease" (p. 19). Being familiar with the impact of historical trauma when conceptualizing issues affecting AI/AN is clearly important.

SUICIDE AMONG AI/AN

The number of AI/AN children and adolescents reporting suicidal ideation is a great cause for concern (Berman, 2006; Olson & Wahab, 2006). In a recent survey of AI/AN adolescents (N = 13,000), 22% of females and 12% of males reported having attempted suicide at some time; 67% who had made an attempt had done so within the past year (Blum, Harmon, Harris, Bergeisen, & Resnick, 1992). In Northwest Alaska, it was found that Eskimo children seen in a community mental health center indicated that previous suicide attempts and substance abuse (including alcohol and inhalant use) were the most common types of problems (Aoun & Gregory, 1998). Since the individual who is at risk for suicide presents a challenging and complex situation that may be difficult to evaluate and difficult to access services for, it is especially important that all AI/AN presenting for medical or mental health services be screened for trauma exposure and potential suicide risk.

DOMESTIC VIOLENCE AND AI/ANS

Domestic violence is a significant concern in AI/AN communities (Evans-Campbell et al., 2006; Harwell et al., 2003; Oetzel & Duran, 2004; Rivers, 2005). There have been recent local and international efforts to understand AI/AN women who have lived through domestic violence (Amnesty International USA, 2007). In addition, while children are often referred to as resilient, it is critical that the real impact of exposure to family violence not be underestimated. Bogat, DeJonghe, Levendosky, Davidson, and von Eye (2006) found a significant relationship between infants (as young as 1-year-olds) and maternal trauma symptoms among those impacted by severe intimate partner violence (IPV). This study demonstrated that even very young children can be impacted by traumatic events, reinforcing the need for early intervention and awareness of domestic violence.

SUBSTANCE ABUSE AND AI/ANs

The literature on substance abuse prevalence and outcomes among AI/AN has been summarized well by several researchers (Szlemko, Wood, & Jumper-Thurman, 2006). American Indian/Alaska Native adolescents have been found to have significant social, psychological, and substance use risk factors (Abbott, 2006). In a recent literature review, Abbott concluded that among American Indian adolescents, there was considerable co-morbidity of psychiatric and substance abuse disorders in the community and clinical populations and that effective screening, early intervention, and treatment programs are needed. While some American Indian residential substance abuse treatment programs exist, many are located miles away from homes, which presents a major barrier to extended family involvement in treatment. Also, since there is some support that caretaker substance use influences adolescent drinking (Walls, Whitbeck, Hoyt, & Johnson, 2007), family-focused treatments are necessary to address the complexities and patterns of problematic substance use.

POST-TRAUMATIC STRESS DISORDER AND AI/AN

Exposure to trauma has been found to be related to risky behaviors, the development of subsequent mental disorders, and PSTD in particular (Kaufman et al., 2004). In a recent study, Kaufman et al. found that trauma plays a role in AI/AN sexual decision-making. In particular, young women who had experienced a trauma had a 20% probability of having multiple casual partners in the prior year compared to 9% for those who have not experienced a trauma (Kaufman et al., 2004). Another study of 89 AI/AN youth in a residential treatment program found that trauma exposure was pervasive: Deters et al. (2006) found an average of 4.1 lifetime traumas among this sample of AI/AN youth, with threat of injury and witnessing injury being the most common form of trauma exposure. It was also found that approximately 10% of participants met the *Diagnostic and Statistical Manual of Mental Disorders* (American Psychiatric Association, 2000) criteria for full PTSD, and about 14% met the criteria for subthreshold PTSD.

TREATMENT ISSUES WITH AI/AN

The degree of cultural competence is a significant issue when working with AI/AN populations. Sue (2006) argues that cultural competency has been largely aspirational (e.g., therapists limiting cultural competency to only the consideration of cultural background or identity of the clients) and needs to move to a "practice-or research-oriented" approach and that "less attention has been given to how cultural competence can be measured, conceptualized in terms of skills, implemented in practice, and trained in others" (Sue, 2006, p. 238). Bernal (2006) has advocated for increased attention to how variables such as values systems (familism, role of spirituality), degree of discrimination, and poverty may impact an individual client and family. LaFromboise, Trimble, and Mohatt (1990) have advocated that the training of American Indian psychologists should move away from conventional tenants of counseling toward the use of culturally sensitive mental health approaches that maintain American Indian values. Gone (2004) has strongly and consistently described the need for change in psychology, and has provided recommendations for "mental health professionals who desire to avoid a subtle but profound Western cultural proselytization in their therapeutic service to native clients and their communities" (Gone, 2004, p. 10). This is an indication of hegemony.

Qualitative studies aimed at understanding the perspectives and experiences of AI/AN have found themes related to traumatic stress and the disconnection of families. For example, in a recent descriptive study with a Pacific Northwest American Indian tribe, Strickland et al. (2006) found that parents and elders wanted to hold the family together and heal intergenerational pains. Recent efforts have been made to provide culturally appropriate mental health services for AI/AN. In 1998, nine AI/AN tribal communities were funded for the Circles of Care (COC) initiative, a collaboration effort of the Center for Mental Health Services of the Substance Abuse and Mental Health Services Administration (SAMHSA), the IHS, and the Office of Juvenile Justice and Delinquency Prevention to provide funding to plan, design, and assess the feasibility of implementing culturally appropriate mental health services for AI/AN children with serious emotional disturbances and their families (Freeman, Iron Cloud-Two Dogs, Novins, & LeMaster, 2004). The COC tribal grantees made extensive efforts to bring attention to the conditions faced by AI/AN through community mobilization and partnerships. Two questions raised by Novins, King, and Stone (2004) throughout the COC planning process were: (a) what constitutes a positive outcome for AI/AN children, adolescents, and their families, and (b) how would these outcomes be measured? These are some of the questions facing many agencies serving AI/AN persons.

EMPIRICALLY SUPPORTED TREATMENTS

Empirically supported treatments (ESTs) are clearly specified psychological treatments shown to be efficacious in controlled research with a delineated population (Chambless & Hollon, 1998). Most current efficacy trials have unknown external validity with respect to the application of ESTs to ethnic minorities (Bernal & Scharron-Del-Rio, 2001). Miranda et al. (2005) reported that American Indian populations are largely missing from the literature on the effectiveness of mental health care and that the limited literature focuses on prevention strategies with American Indian youth. Bernal and Scharron-Del-Rio suggest that "it is essential that researchers construct theories of psychotherapy and evaluate treatments grounded in the realities and experiences of ethnic minority populations" (2001, p. 337). In addition, Bernal and Saez-Santiago (2006) reported that too few studies have: (a) incorporated culture and ethnicity as part of the intervention; (b) tested the effectiveness of such interventions; (c) articulated and documented how ethnicity and culture play a role in the treatment process; and (d) described how interventions may need to be adapted or tailored to meet the needs of diverse families.[3]

A recent article by Miranda et al. (2005) identified interventions for Latino, Puerto Rican, and African-American populations. However, no studies evaluating outcomes of mental health care for AI/AN were found. Although conceptual in nature, Coteau, Anderson, and Hope (2006) took a needed step forward by highlighting some of the unique challenges of adapting manualized anxiety treatments with AI/AN, while Whitbeck (2006) has identified a five-stage model for developing evidence-based culturally specific intervention and assessment models with AIs. The stages include the need to: (a) be familiar with key risk factors and protective factors that European prevention researchers bring to the prevention effort; (b) be familiar with previous culturally specific research that has been done with the particular culture; (c) work with cultural experts to adapt or "translate" key risk and protective factors to fit the cultural context; (d) develop measures of risk and protective factors that may be unique to the culture; and (e) conduct culturally specific intervention trials and assessments.

ADAPTATION OF EVIDENCE-BASED PRACTICES FOR AI/AN

Evidence-based practice (EBP) is the integration of the best available research with clinical expertise in the context of patient characteristics, culture, and preferences (American Psychological Association Presidential Task Force on Evidence-Based Practice, 2006) and is a broader concept than ESTs. It has been suggested that treatments that are straightforward and easier to learn are more likely to be disseminated to the larger practice community (Chambless & Hollon, 1998). The National Institute of Mental Health's (1999) strategic plan for reducing health disparities pointed out that "scientifically proven interventions must be disseminated to the clinics, schools, and other places where children, adolescents, and their parents can easily access them" (1999, p. 6). The Indian Country Child Trauma Center (ICCTC), at the University of Oklahoma Health Sciences Center, is working with the NCTSN and SAMHSA to develop, refine, disseminate, and evaluate culturally relevant trauma intervention models and protocols for use with children in Indian Country. The ICCTC (2006) has identified a set of empirically supported child trauma intervention models and has built on the foundation of AI/AN traditional teachings and practices to develop culturally relevant treatment interventions. The premise of the cultural adaptation is the belief that AI/AN cultures have current healing practices, activities, and ceremonies that were and are used therapeutically and are based on knowing how to instruct individuals regarding relationships, children, and parenting.

The process of adaptation led by ICCTC faculty parallel and expands the recommendations of Whitbeck (2006) and included other aspects learned from implementation of their Project Making Medicine training (Project Making Medicine, 2005). The process for adaptation included: (a) reviewing the core components of EBP, including trauma focused-cognitive behavioral therapy (see Figure 1), treatment of children with

FIGURE 1. Native Adaptations for Trauma Focused-Cognitive Behavioral Therapy.

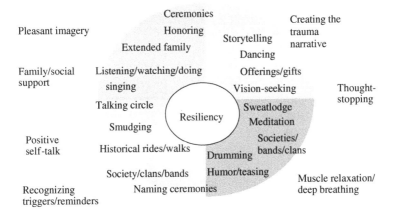

sexual behavioral problems, and parent-child interaction therapy; (b) reviewing the current counseling research literature with AI/AN and working with the original developers to make adaptations; (c) cultural consultants were identified, met on the process and content of the cultural adaptations, and provided on-going feedback, along with feedback from practitioners and community members; and (d) adaptations (removal and addition) of information to the original EBP being done. Three evidence-based treatments by ICCTC were created: *Honoring Children, Mending the Circle* (BigFoot & Schmidt, 2006), *Honoring Children, Respectful Ways* (Silovsky, Burris, McElroy, BigFoot, & Bonner, 2005), and *Honoring Children, Making Relatives* (Funderburk, Gurwitch, & BigFoot, 2005). In addition, the ICCTC developed a suicide intervention/prevention component called *Honoring Children, Honoring the Future*. Additional lessons learned from the efforts to adapt and implement evidence-based treatments are the need for program and administration support; collective training of critical supervisors and clinicians; ongoing consultation; and the development of an implementation that includes evaluation plus institutionalization of the model.[4]

LOOKING TOWARD THE FUTURE

American Indian/Alaska Natives are establishing local programs to promote well-being that is culturally congruent within their community settings. Local consortiums that include tribal colleges have been the leaders in developing and establishing pathways for healthier living and decreasing violence by teaching and training in advocacy and community mobilization. Tribal colleges are taking their role seriously to increase the capacity of communities by providing courses in mental health as well as being innovators in developing services.[5]

Other efforts to promote culturally congruent services include work done by White Bison (www.whitebison.org) through their Sacred Hoop Journeys and Wellbriety Movements, offering sobriety, recovery, addictions and violence prevention, and wellness resources; the Sacred Circle National Resource Center to End Violence Against Women (www.sacredcircle.com/), committed to community mobilization and increasing awareness on the harm toward AI/AN women and children, has brought international attention to violence against AI/AN; and the First Nations Behavioral Health (http://www.fnbha.org), which advocates for the mental well-being of Native peoples by increasing the knowledge and awareness of issues impacting Native mental health, has provided national leadership on creating collaborative, culturally congruent, community-based services.

Recent efforts supported by SAMSHA and tribal entities and organizations such as the National Congress of American Indians (www.ncai.org/), IHS (www.ihs.gov), and the Bureau of Indian Affairs have created opportunities for proactive strategizing at the community level for coalition building and community ownership. Tribal members are the critical decision-makers to make lasting changes in addressing issues of substance abuse, violence, and mental health (see www.NICWA.org). Realizing that it takes more than a mental health provider to impact communities, community coalitions are committed to addressing systems change (e.g., infrastructure in tribal communities) and involving the community in research (e.g., participatory-based research). These efforts will have a lasting impact on the mental healthcare provided to AI/AN children and families.

SUMMARY

This article sought to share how violence and the resulting trauma has had a major impact on AI/AN children and their families, creating hardships that have been very difficult to address or overcome. The recent published literature on poverty and historical trauma provides a contextual framework for understanding issues of violence and the resulting trauma, suicide, domestic violence, and PTSD shared by many AI/AN communities. Cultural adaptations of evidence-based treatments (see Chamberlain, 2008, this issue) are one attempt to integrate Western psychology with indigenous ways of the knowing. Indigenous people are seeking to regain their healing ways by looking around their circle and drawing toward them ways that work and ways to address violence.

NOTES

1. American Indian and Alaska Native are terminology to designate the indigenous people of the United States with the following terms used interchangeably with tribes, native, native people, and indigenous people.

2. More information about tribal groups can be found at the *Encyclopedia Smithsonian*, available from www.si.edu/Encyclopedia_SI/History_and_Culture/AmericanIndian_History.htm

3. For a more detailed discussion, see the National Mental Health Council's Clinical Treatment and Services Research Workgroup (2000).

4. More information about the adapted models can be found at www.icctc.org.

5. See *Tribal College Journal of American Indian Education* at www.tribalcollegejo urnal.org/

REFERENCES

Abbott, P. J. (2006). Co-morbid alcohol/other drug abuse/dependence and psychiatric disorders in adolescent American Indian and Alaska Natives. *Alcoholism Treatment Quarterly, 24*(4), 3–21.

American Psychiatric Association (APA). (2000). *Diagnostic and statistical manual of mental disorders* (4th ed.). Washington, DC: Author.

American Psychological Association Presidential Task Force on Evidence-Based Practice. (2006, May–June). Evidence-based practice in psychology. *American Psychologist, 61*(4), 271–285.

Amnesty International USA. (2007). *Maze of injustice: The failure of protect indigenous women from sexual violence in the USA.* Retrieved September 13, 2007, from http://www.amnestyusa.org/women/maze/report.pdf

Aoun, S. L., & Gregory, R. J. (1998). Mental disorders of Eskimos who were seen at a community mental health center in western Alaska. *Psychiatric Services, 49,* 1485–1487.

Berman, A. L. (2006). Risk management with suicidal patients. *Journal of Clinical Psychology, 62,* 171–184.

Bernal, G. (2006). Intervention development and cultural adaptation research with diverse families. *Family Process, 45*(2), 143–151.

Bernal, G., & Saez-Santiago, E. (2006). Culturally centered psychosocial interventions. *Journal of Community Psychology, 34*(2), 121–132.

Bernal, G., & Scharron-Del-Rio, M. R. (2001). Are empirically supported treatments valid for ethnic minorities? Toward an alternative approach for treatment research. *Cultural Diversity and Ethnic Minority Psychology, 7*(4), 328–342.

BigFoot, D. S. (1989). Parenting training for American Indian families. *Dissertation Abstracts International, 50*(6), 1562A.

BigFoot, D. S. (2000). History of victimization in Native communities. In D. BigFoot (Ed.), *Native American topic-specific monograph series.* Washington DC: Office for Victims of Crime.

BigFoot, D. S., & Braden, J. (2007). Adapting evidence-based treatments for use with American Indian and Native Alaska children and youth. *Focal Point, 21*(1), 19–22.

BigFoot, D. S., & Schmidt, S. (2006). *Honoring children, mending the circle (trauma-focused cognitive behavior therapy).* Indian Country Child Trauma Center, University of Oklahoma Health Sciences Center, Oklahoma City, OK.

Blum, R. W., Harmon, B., Harris, L., Bergeisen, L., & Resnick, M. D. (1992). American Indian-Alaska Native youth health. *Journal of the American Medical Association, 267,* 1637–1644.

Bogat, G. A., DeJonghe, E., Levendosky, A. A., Davidson, W. S., & von Eye, A. (2006). Trauma symptoms among infants exposed to intimate partner violence. *Child Abuse & Neglect, 30*, 109–125.

Bouman, J. (2006). *What the census should say.* Retrieved September 18, 2007, from http://www.dmiblog.com/archives/2006/08/what_the_census_should_say.html.

Chamberlain, L. (2008). Ten lessons learned in Alaska: Home visitation and intimate partner violence. *Journal of Emotional Abuse, 8*(1/2), 205–216.

Chambless, D. L., & Hollon, S. D. (1998). Defining empirically supported therapies. *Journal of Consulting and Clinical Psychology, 66*(1), 7–18.

Cohen, J. A., Mannarino, A. P., & Deblinger, E. (2006). *Treating trauma and traumatic grief in children and adolescents.* New York: The Guilford Press.

Cole, N. (2006). Trauma and the American Indian. In T. M. Witko (Ed.), *Mental health care for urban Indians: Clinical insights from Native practitioners* (pp. 115–130). Washington DC: American Psychological Association.

Colmant, S., Schultz, L., Robbins, R., Ciali, P., Dorton, J., & Rivera-Colmant, Y. (2004). Constructing meaning to the Indian boarding school experience. *Journal of American Indian Education, 43*(3), 22–40.

Coteau, T. D., Anderson, J., & Hope, D. (2006). Adapting manualized treatments. Treating anxiety disorders among Native Americans. *Cognitive and Behavioral Practice, 13*, 304–309.

Deters, P. B., Novins, D. K., Fickenscher, A., & Beals, J. (2006). Trauma and posttraumatic stress disorder symptomatology: Patterns among American Indian adolescents in substance abuse treatment. *American Journal of Orthopsychiatry, 76*(3), 335–345.

Duran, E. (2006). *Healing the soul wound: Counseling with American Indians and other native peoples.* New York: Teachers College Press.

Ehlers, C. L., Hurst, S., Phillips, E., Gilder, D. A., Dixon, M., Gross, A., et al. (2006). Electrophysiological responses to affective stimuli in American Indians experiencing trauma with and without PTSD. *Annals New York Academy of Sciences, 1071*, 125–136.

Evans-Campbell, T., Lindhorst, T., Huang, B., & Walters, K. L. (2006). Interpersonal violence in the lives of urban American Indian and Alaska Native women: Implications for health, mental health, and help-seeking. *American Journal of Public Health, 96*, 1416–1422.

Freeman, B., Iron Cloud-Two Dogs, E., Novins, D., & LeMaster, P. L. (2004). Contextual issues for strategic planning and evaluation of systems of care for American Indian and Alaska Native communities: An introduction to Circles of Care. *American Indian and Alaska Native Mental Health Research, 11*(2), 1–29.

Fuller-Thomson, E., & Minkler, M. (2005). American Indian/Alaska native grandparents raising grandchildren: Findings from the Census 2000 Supplemental Survey. *NASW*, 131–139.

Funderburk, B. W., Gurwitch, R., & BigFoot, D. S. (2005) *Honoring children, making relatives: Parent child interaction therapy training manual.* Indian Country Child Trauma Center, University of Oklahoma Health Sciences Center, Oklahoma City, OK.

Garrett, M. T., Garrett, J. T., & Brotherton, D. (2001). Inner circle/outer circle: A group technique based on Native American healing circles. *Journal for Specialists in Group Work, 26*(1), 17–30.

Gone, J. P. (2004). Mental health services for Native Americans in the 21st century United States. *Professional Psychology: Research and Practice, 35*(1), 10–18.

Harwell, T. S., Moore, K. R., & Spence, M. R. (2003). Physical violence, intimate partner violence, and emotional abuse among adult American Indian men and women in Montana. *Preventive Medicine, 37*, 297–303.

Hill, D. L. (2006). Sense of belonging as connectedness, American Indian worldview, and mental health. *Archives of Psychiatric Nursing, 20*(5), 210–216.

House, L. E., Stiffman, A. R., & Brown, E. (2006). Unraveling cultural threads: A qualitative study of culture and ethnic identity among urban southwestern American Indian youth, parents, and elders. *Journal of Child and Family Studies, 15*(4), 393–407.

Indian Country Child Trauma Center. (2006). University of Oklahoma Health Sciences Center. Retrieved February 16, 2007, from www.icctc.org.

Kaufman, C. E., Beals, J., Mitchell, C. M., LeMaster, P., & Fickenscher, A. (2004). Stress, trauma, and risky sexual behaviour among American Indians in young adulthood. *Culture, Health & Sexuality, 6*(4), 301–318.

La Fromboise, T. D., & Heyle, A.M. (1990). Changing and diverse roles of women in American Indian cultures. *Sex Roles, 22*, 455–476.

La Fromboise, T. D., Trimble, J. E., & Mohatt, G. V. (1990). Counseling intervention and American Indian tradition: An integrative approach. *The Counseling Psychologist, 18*(4), 628–654.

McCabe, G. H. (2007). The healing path: A culture and community-derived indigenous therapy model. *Psychotherapy: Theory, Research, Practice, Training, 44*(2), 148–160.

Miranda, J., Bernal, G., Lau, A., Kohn, L., Hwang, W., & La Fromboise, T. (2005). State of the science on psychosocial interventions for ethnic minorities. *Annual Review of Clinical Psychology, 1*, 113–142.

National Mental Health Council's Clinical Treatment and Services Research Workgroup. (2000). *Translating behavioral science into action* (NIH Publication No. 00–4699). Rockville, MD: National Institute on Mental Health.

National Child Abuse and Neglect Data System. (2002). *Child abuse and neglect statistics.* Retrieved February 16, 2007, from http://www.childwelfare.gov/systemwide/statistics/can.cfm.

National Child Traumatic Stress Network. (2005). *Trauma.* Retrieved February 16, 2007, from www.nctsn.org

National Insitute of Mental Health. (1999). *Strategic plan on reducing health disparities* (draft). Rockville, MD: Author.

Novins, D. K., King, M., & Stone, L. S. (2004). Developing a plan for measuring outcomes in model systems of care for American Indian and Alaska Native children and youth. *American Indian & Alaska Native Mental Health Research, 11*(2), 88–96.

Oetzel, J., & Duran, B. (2004). Intimate partner violence in American Indian and/or Alaska Native communities: A social ecological framework of determinants and interventions. *American Indian & Alaska Native Mental Health Research, 11*, 49–68.

Ogunwole, S. U. (2002, February). *The American Indian and Alaska Native population: 2000.* Retrieved September 13, 2007, from http://www.census.gov.

Olson, L. M., & Wahab, S. (2006). American Indians and suicide: A neglected area of research. *Trauma, Violence, & Abuse, 7*(1), 19–33.

Project Making Medicine. (2005). *Project Making Medicine Final Report.* Oklahoma City, OK: University of Oklahoma Health Sciences Center to Indian Health Service.

Rivers, M. J. (2005). Navajo women and abuse: The context for their troubled relationships. *Journal of Family Violence, 20,* 83–89.

Silovsky, J. F., Burris, L. J., McElroy, E., BigFoot, D. S., & Bonner, B. L. (2005) *Honoring children, respectful ways: Treatment for Native children with sexual behavior problems.* Indian Country Child Trauma Center, University of Oklahoma Health Sciences Center, Oklahoma City, OK.

Stannard, D. E. (1992). *American holocaust.* New York: Oxford University Press.

Strickland, C. J., Walsh, E., & Cooper, M. (2006). Healing fractured families: Parents' and Elders' perspectives on the impact of colonization and youth suicide prevention in a Pacific Northwest American Indian tribe. *Journal of Transcultural Nursing, 17*(1), 5–12.

Sue, S. (2006). Cultural competency: From philosophy to research and practice. *Journal of Community Psychology, 34*(2), 237–245.

Szlemko, W. J., Wood, J. W., & Jumper-Thurman, P. (2006). Native Americans and alcohol: Past, present, and future. *The Journal of General Psychology, 133*(4), 435–451.

U.S. Census Bureau. (2000). American Indian/Alaska Native data and links. Retrieved February 16, 2007, from http://factfinder.census.gov/home/aian/index.html.

Walls, M. L., Whitbeck, L. B., Hoyt, D. R., & Johnson, K. D. (2007, May). Early-onset alcohol use among Native American youth: Examining female caretaker influence. *Journal of Marriage and Family, 69,* 451–464.

Weaver, H. N. (1998). Indigenous people in a multicultural society: Unique issues for human services. *Social Work, 43*(3), 203- 211.

Whitbeck, L. B. (2006). Some guiding assumptions and a theoretical model for developing culturally specific preventions with Native American people. *Journal of Community Psychology, 34*(2), 183–192.

Zuckerman, S., Haley, J. M., Roubideaux, Y., & Lillie-Blanton, M. (2004). Access, use, and insurance coverage among American Indians/Alaska Natives and Whites: What role does the Indian Health Service play? *American Journal Public Health, 94,* 53–59.

Proximity and Risk in Children's Witnessing of Intimate Partner Violence Incidents

Abigail H. Gewirtz
Amanuel Medhanie

The past two decades have seen an upsurge of interest in documenting and understanding children's witnessing of intimate partner violence (IPV; e.g., Cicchetti & Toth, 1995; Edleson, 1999; Geffner, Jaffe, & Sudermann, 2000; Gewirtz & Edleson, 2007; Margolin & Gordis, 2000). In particular, studies examining the prevalence, incidence, and impact of exposure to violence on development have resulted in efforts to develop and document early interventions for child witnesses (Berkowitz, 2003; Cohen, 2003; Gewirtz, Harris, & Avendano, 2006). A key challenge for the field is to gather information on event parameters, children's experiences, and reactions during and immediately after a traumatic event. Such information is more readily accessible for events occurring in the community than for violence occurring within homes, which is often underreported (Straus & Gelles, 1990). Hence, not surprisingly, there is a dearth of data regarding contextual or incident details and children's responses during and soon after exposure to IPV (see Kracke & Hahn, 2008, this issue). Much of the research on children's exposure to IPV focuses on the relationship between exposure and children's functioning months to years after the violent event or events (McCloskey, Figueredo, & Koss, 1995; McCloskey & Walker, 2000; O'Brien, John, Margolin, & Erel, 1994; Zuckerman, Augustyn, Groves, & Parker, 1995), with little focus on the details of single events or shorter time periods (an exception is Jouriles et al., 1998). Although such data offer "big picture" information, there are few studies that provide basic descriptive information about children in the context of single violent incidents: their involvement, proximity, acute adjustment, and other descriptive information (Ernst, Weiss, & Enright-Smith, 2006; Fantuzzo, Boruch, Beriama, Atkins, & Marcus, 1997). This article contributes to the current literature on children's exposure to IPV and acute traumatic stressors by providing key descriptive details about the nature, proximity, and parameters of children's involvement as witnesses to IPV, and their variation by age, gender, and family relationships. In addition, this is the first article that we know of that provides concurrent data on acute risk and functioning in the immediate aftermath of an incident of IPV.

The lack of information on children's experiences in IPV incidents is not surprising (see Kracke & Cohen, 2008, this issue). First, the underreporting of children's involvement in IPV incidents has been amply documented (e.g., Bachman & Coker, 1995; Edleson, Mbilinyi, Beeman, & Hagemeister, 2003; Mihalic & Elliott, 1997). Several authors have documented parents' underestimation of the extent of children's witnessing of violent incidents even as their children describe details of events they were not supposed to have seen (e.g., Edleson, 1999; Jaffe, Wolfe, & Wilson, 1990). This underreporting may be due, in part, to policies in some jurisdictions that mandate the reporting to child protective agencies of incidents where children are actively involved in IPV.[1] Second, the acute nature of violent events precludes the use of standard research designs to elicit information about children's experiences and involvement during violent events (Edleson et al., 2003). Third, despite increasing interest in the investigation and prosecution of IPV incidents, particularly those involving children (Gewirtz, Miller, Weidner, & Zehm, 2006), most police departments do not routinely mandate documenting the presence of children in an officer's police reports. Hence, many child witnesses to IPV are, literally, "invisible" to official documentation (Osofsky, 1997; Rosenbaum & O'Leary, 1981). Finally, the lack of a formal classification system or national surveillance system for children's exposure to IPV precludes gathering national epidemiological data on the extent and range of children's experiences with regard to IPV compared with, for example, child abuse and neglect experiences (see concerns regarding definitions in Kracke & Hahn, 2008, this issue).

Despite these drawbacks, multi-informant data on IPV incidents, when available, can be extremely useful for understanding children's involvement. Sources of information may include parent report, child self-report, other witness report and/or police report (when such incidents are reported to police, and when police document child witness details). When police are called, police reports can be key sources of information about event parameters, physical evidence, witness descriptions, and children's involvement at the scene of an IPV incident. For example, in their description of children's witnessing of IPV through the Spousal Abuse Replication Study (SARP), Fantuzzo et al. (1997) used police reports and victim interviews to describe children's involvement in misdemeanor IPV incidents in five cities. Findings indicated that children under 5 were disproportionately involved in IPV incidents, and that there was a range of child involvement, including child calls to 911. However, the study did not track details of children's exposure to violence or developmental differences in children's exposure.

Knowledge of children's event-related experiences and functioning during and immediately after IPV incidents is critical in the following ways: (a) to provide details that can further delineate the similarities and differences in children's reactions to varied traumatic stressors; (b) because event/exposure characteristics have consistently been identified as significant predictors of recovery and adjustment in both the short and longer term aftermath of traumatic events (e.g., La Greca, Silverman, Vernberg, & Prinstein, 1996; Pine & Cohen, 2002), and hence are important for the development of early preventive interventions for such children; and (c) because context- or incident-specific details of violent events can also help to further our understanding of specificity in the relationship between witnessing violence and adjustment outcomes (McMahon, Grant, Compas, Thurm, & Ey, 2003).

RISK AND CHILD ADJUSTMENT FOLLOWING VIOLENT INCIDENTS

Several factors have been identified as important in understanding recovery and adjustment among traumatized children (Green, Korol, & Grace, 1991; Chamberlain, 2008, this issue; La Greca et al., 1996; Pine & Cohen, 2002). These include event parameters (details of the event and the child's involvement, particularly, degree of exposure to the traumatic event), individual child risk and protective factors (e.g., history of trauma, psychopathology, and socio-demographics), and environmental variables (e.g., parental reactions, social and parental support of the child, etc.).

For all types of trauma, the level of exposure to the event has consistently predicted the later level of psychopathology (Pine & Cohen, 2002). This has been documented more clearly in studies of disaster and community violence (see Kracke & Hahn, 2008, this issue), such as in a study of a school shooting that indicated that children who were more proximal to the sniper or who visually witnessed the event were more likely to manifest subsequent traumatic stress symptoms (Nader, Pynoos, Fairbanks, & Frederick, 1990; Pynoos & Nader, 1989).

Developmental psychopathology approaches to the study of stress and adversity in development have emphasized the vulnerability to subsequent adjustment associated with children's experience of prior trauma events

(Cicchetti & Toth, 1995). For example, McCloskey and Walker (2000), in a sample of 237 school-age children, found that prior trauma experiences (i.e., child abuse, domestic violence, and death or illness of a close family member) were predisposing factors for post-traumatic stress disorder. We could find no studies, however, that investigated the relationship between prior or event-related risk and children's concurrent adjustment in the near aftermath of a violent incident. Such data would be important for understanding the determinants of recovery among traumatized children, and in particular, the development of a comprehensive model of post-trauma functioning that takes into account the relationships between prior risks, event-related risks, functioning shortly after a traumatic event, and subsequent disorder in the months following.

The goals of the current study were (a) to gather basic descriptive details of children's participation in violent incidents and (b) to understand predictors of child functioning soon after the incident. Data were analyzed from an existing data set that provided a combination of police, clinician, and self-report data about child witnesses to IPV incidents resulting in 911 calls.

Research Questions

1. What is the nature and extent of children's involvement in IPV incidents? Are there developmental and/or gender differences in involvement in violent incidents?
2. Do a combination of acute (i.e., proximity) and chronic risks (i.e., prior trauma exposure) predict child functioning within the days following a violent incident?

METHOD

Sample

Data for this study were gathered from the records of the Minneapolis Child Development Policing Program (CDPP). The CDPP is a multidisciplinary community-university partnership aimed at providing acute clinical and advocacy services to children and families following their exposure to violence. The purpose of the program is to increase access to care for children exposed to violence and ultimately to ameliorate the impact of violence on children's development and adjustment. The program, which is voluntary for families, is a partnership of police officers and mental health professionals who respond jointly, as soon as possible after a violent incident,[2] to offer acute services to families with children who have called 911 for IPV. Clinicians provide psycho-education for parents about the impact of exposure to violence on children, assessment and referral to a broad range of social services, and crisis de-escalation with cognitive-behavioral techniques. Police officers provide information about the investigation and criminal justice process. Cases were referred to the team by the commander of the Family Violence Unit at the Minneapolis Police Department, who reviewed all prior-week family violence cases and referred all those cases involving children.

Following receipt of Institutional Review Board approval, we reviewed police reports and program records of 818 cases referred to the CDPP intervention program from April 2003 until April 2005. Criteria for inclusion in the final sample analyzed included: (a) basic information about the case was available (i.e., a police report existed, plus some service record documentation); (b) precipitating incident was adult intimate partner violence; and (c) this was a family's first referral to CDPP. Three hundred and eleven families were excluded from the final sample because they were referred for other presenting incidents (e.g., community violence exposure, mental health difficulties, the child was the alleged perpetrator), because the case involved a family already in the database, or because insufficient documentation was available for analysis. The final sample included 507 families with 1012 children.

Police report data included details of the incident (as noted on the police report), information about the child(ren's) presence and involvement in the incident, and demographic information on the victim, perpetrator, and child witnesses. Clinical service records captured a wide range of information about children and families, but the amount and depth of information collected varied widely, depending upon the length and nature of the contact with the clinical team. For example, cases involved no contact (family was out when the CDPP team visited) to meetings with the family (lasting 5 minutes to 1.5 hours), and children were not always present during the CDPP team visits. When clinicians had direct, more extended contact with both child(ren) and family (at least 30 minutes), clinicians completed a clinical assessment, including ratings of child behavior and a global assessment of child functioning (Child Global Assessment Scale (CGAS); Schaffer et al., 1983), based upon knowledge gathered in the course of the interview with child and family and observations of the child.

Measures

For this study, we utilized data from both police[3] and clinical service records. Data gathered from police reports included: child age, race, and gender; relationship of child to victim and perpetrator; relationship between victim and perpetrator; number of children in the family; and details of the incident and of the child's proximity to the violent event. Information about each child's proximity to the violent event was culled from the descriptive information on the police reports and rated by the research team on a four point scale: "not in home," "present in home, but asleep or not in same room/indirect witnessing," "direct witnessing (in same room)," and "direct involvement in violence" (e.g., physically hurt, intervened in the violence, made 911 call, etc.). Additional data gathered from the police report included the elements of the incident (whether or not the incident included the use of a weapon, physical assault, verbal abuse, and/or property damage). Data gathered from the clinical service record included the number of days between the incident and the CDPP intervention (i.e., the team's visit), and for the subsample of children for whom data regarding psychological functioning were available, clinician-rated CGAS data were accessed. The CGAS (Schaffer et al., 1983) provides a global measure of functioning in children and adolescents, on a scale of 0–100, with the measure's glossary details determining the meaning of the points on the scale. Clinicians were instructed to rate the child's most impaired level of functioning for the time period they were present with the child. The clinical team also gathered data from the child's caregiver about the child's prior trauma history, including whether or not the child had experienced prior death or serious illness of a parent, removal to foster care placement, and/or physical assault or intentional injury.

Descriptive Statistics

The sample consisted of 507 families with 1012 children, for whom more detailed socio-demographic data were available for 874 children. Children's mean age was 7.11, with half of the children age 6 years or younger. There were almost equal numbers of boys and girls (50.9% females, 49.1% boys), but boys were significantly younger than girls (7.03 vs. 7.94), $t(766) = 2.51$, $p = .012$. The mean and median number of children in each household was two, although the range of children in each household was one to eight. The vast majority of the sample comprised children of color, with 63% African-American; 12% Caucasian; 7% Hispanic; 4% Native American; 10% bi- or multi-racial; 1% African; 1% Asian; and 2% other. More than half of the children (54%) were the biological offspring of both victim and perpetrator; 87% children were the biological offspring of the victim.

Of the 507 cases reviewed, the vast majority of incidents involved physical aggression (83%), with verbal abuse present in 68% of incidents and property destruction an element of almost one-quarter of the cases (24%). A weapon (a knife or a gun) was used in 15% of the cases. Drugs or alcohol were described on the police report to be a factor in 87.5% of the cases. Prior IPV (reported either by the adult or on the police report) was reported in 69% of the cases. Proximity data were available for 635 children in 390 families. Fourteen percent of children were not present in the home at the time of the incident, 16% were indirectly exposed (i.e., did not visually witness the incident but were in the home at the time of the incident), 57% were direct witnesses to the violence, and 12% were directly involved in the violence (e.g., by dialing 911, attempting to prevent the assault, or being physically assaulted themselves).

In order to investigate the relationship between proximity and child functioning, we analyzed data from a subset of the larger sample of 507 families. This subsample ($N = 66$ children) represented the first child noted in the clinical record from each of 66 families for whom CGAS data were available. There were no significant differences between the subsample and the larger sample (minus the subsample) on child's age ($M = 7.36$ vs. 7.05), $t(451) = -0.459$, $p = 0.64$; race (minority vs. nonminority), $\chi^2(1, N = 422) = 0.386$, $p = 0.11$; gender, $\chi^2(1, N = 423) = 0.45$, $p = 0.50$; number of children in the family ($M = 2.18$ vs. 1.97), $t(505) = 1.39$, $p = 0.16$; relationship of the target child to the victim, $\chi^2(8, N = 763) = 10.61$, $p = 0.23$; the child's proximity to the event, $\chi^2(1, N = 334) = 5.38$, 3, $p = 0.15$; substance use involvement in the incident (87% vs. 87.6%), $\chi^2(1, N = 176) = 0.00$, $p = 0.93$; and prior report of IPV (83.1% vs. 66.8%), $\chi^2(1, N = 420) = 6.87$, $p = 0.11$.

RESULTS

Patterns of Children's Proximity to Violent Incidents

Children's proximity patterns were analyzed for three categories of proximity: indirect exposure, direct witness, and direct involvement (Children who were not present in the home during the incident [$N = 91$] were removed from this analysis.). The mean age of children who were indirectly involved was 6.12 ($SD = 5.03$), mean age of direct witnesses was 7.31 ($SD = 4.8$), and mean age of children with direct involvement was 9.05 ($SD = 5.6$). A one-way analysis of variance with child's proximity as the independent variable (three categories) and age as the dependent variable revealed a significant difference between mean ages by proximity, $F(2, 506) = 7.55$; $p = .001$.

The significant positive relationship between age and proximity to violence held up for both genders separately. However, although the overall equation was significant among boys, there was no difference in average age between those indirectly exposed ($M = 6.50$ years) and direct witnesses ($M = 6.50$ years), whereas boys who were physically involved were significantly older ($M = 9.05$ years). Among girls, a more even spread across age was evident (M age for indirect exposure = 6.56; for direct exposure = 8.27; for physically involved = 9.42).

Age and Weapons

We conducted a two-sample *t*-test to investigate the relationship between age and presence or absence of a weapon. The results revealed that children who witnessed incidents involving guns or knives were significantly older than those who witnessed incidents that did not involve weapons ($M = 7.92$ vs. 6.94), $t(872) = -2.20$, $p = 0.03$.

Proximity, Prior Trauma History, and Child Adjustment

We predicted that children's functioning in the few days after exposure to a violent incident would be partly predicted by time since the incident (i.e., the more days since the incident, the better the child's functioning), as well as by a combination of acute and chronic risks: the child's proximity to the incident, and the child's prior trauma history. In order to examine the contributions of the acute and prior risk variables on CGAS, proximity (two levels: indirect witness or not present vs. direct witness or physical involvement), prior trauma (two levels: yes/no), and number of days since the incident (i.e., number of days between the incident and the visit) were entered into a regression equation. Table 1 indicates that the

TABLE 1. Linear regression analysis predicting CGAS ($N = 61$)[4]

Variable	B	SE B	β
Days after incident	.901	.699	.162
Evidence of past trauma history	−5.53	3.75	−.19
Proximity (two categories)	−7.46	4.57	−.20

Model $R^2 = .12$; $p = .06$.

overall equation approached significance at $p = .06$, with the overall model accounting for 12.1% of the variance in children's psychological functioning, although none of the independent variables separately reached significance.

DISCUSSION

In this study of families calling 911 for emergency services for IPV, we were able to delineate patterns in children's exposure to IPV incidents. Most children living in the home were direct witnesses to the violent incident (i.e., they visually witnessed and/or were directly involved in the incident), consistent with prior studies that have utilized police reports (e.g., Ernst et al., 2006; Fantuzzo et al., 1997). Moreover, children's proximity to the violent event was associated with age, such that older children were more likely to be present and involved in the violent incident. In particular, among both boys and girls, direct involvement in the violent incident (e.g., by calling 911 or physically intervening) was positively associated with older age. Analyses also uncovered a significant positive association between children's age and the use of a weapon during a violent incident: older children were more likely to be present during incidents involving weapons.

We could find no prior studies examining the relationship between children's age and proximity or roles during violent incidents. However, the findings are consistent with accounts of the impact of development on children's perceptions of their roles in violent incidents (Groves, 2003; Marans & Adelman, 1997; Osofsky, 2003). Thus, as children of both genders age, they may feel increasingly compelled to intervene in some way on behalf of a victimized caregiver. Indeed, the clinical experiences of the CDPP clinicians reflect our findings. For example, the CDPP team visited a family where, during an incident in which a man physically assaulted his wife, their 9-year-old daughter had thrown a shoe at her father in an attempt to stop him. In response, her father shoved the girl away, and the girl fled the room and placed a 911 call. The CDPP team visited the family a day later. During the visit, the girl reported to the clinician and officer that she had witnessed ongoing IPV over the past several years and finally decided that the time had come for her to help her mother. The findings of a significant association between age and proximity suggests that safety planning for children should be a key element in acute intervention programs.

In this study, the "direct involvement" category of proximity included both actual physical involvement in the violence and involvement that may be nonphysical (e.g., placing a 911 call). Accordingly, the range of danger presented by the child's involvement varies according to the situation, the child's age, and the type of involvement of the child. For example, for a school-aged child, attempting to break up a fight is generally more dangerous than placing a 911 call (particularly if the child has fled to a neighbor to do so). Further research should examine the details of children's physical involvement in violence, for example, by categorizing whether the involvement was escape/help-oriented (e.g., 911 call) or defensive/aggressively oriented (i.e., intervening to attack the abuser, to protect the victim, or stop the assault).

The finding of a significant association between age and weapon also presents further questions. It is unclear why the likelihood of being present at an incident involving a weapon increases with a child's age. However, successful replications of this finding would suggest that clinical interventions with older school age children should focus not only on safety planning per se, but specifically on safety planning in the subcategory of violent incidents involving guns or knives.

Beyond descriptions of the role of children who witness IPV incidents, we also analyzed the impact of incident-related and prior trauma experiences on the child's functioning at the time of the clinician-officer visit. A regression analysis indicated that the combination of current and prior trauma risks approached significance in their prediction of the child's functioning during the clinician visit. These results must be interpreted cautiously, as the sample size is small, and the significance is marginal at $p = .06$. However, this is the first study that we know of to investigate the relationship between prior trauma, event-related risks, and children's functioning shortly after a violent event. From a clinical perspective, the data imply that those providing services to children in post-traumatic circumstances should take a broad view of the child's situation by considering the child's historical and current risks. From a research perspective, these data suggest the need to develop more complex models to predict children's functioning immediately after violent events. Such models would incorporate measures of event-related, prior trauma history, and socio-demographic risk and protective factors in accounting for post-traumatic functioning in children.

LIMITATIONS

This study utilized data gathered in the course of a crisis intervention program. As such, the measures were constrained by the emergency contexts in which they were gathered, and lacked the depth or details that would be preferable in measuring variables such as functioning or trauma history. Similarly, the use of standardized tools with established reliability and validity would have increased the generalizability of our findings.

In addition, the data were derived from reports of families who called the police for IPV and these families represent but a subset of families who experience IPV. For example, Bachman and Coker (1995) have documented that African-American women are more likely than White women to call the police following an IPV incident. Our data are obviously limited to those families who have called the police, and may also overrepresent families of color. More research is needed with larger samples in order to comprehensively examine the relationship between acute and prior risk variables and children's functioning following IPV incidents.

CONCLUSIONS

This study contributes important details to understanding risk factors in children's witnessing of IPV incidents. Fantuzzo and colleagues (1997) noted that "research on children who witness family violence is a special case of counting the hard-to-count and measuring the hard-to-measure" (p. 121). In this study, we tried to measure the "hard-to-measure" by accessing data from a police-mental health intervention for children who have recently witnessed IPV. These data provide a basis for further research that is needed to develop a comprehensive model of risk and protective factors for children who are exposed to violent incidents.

A key question for the field is the appropriate timing and nature of early interventions for children exposed to violence (Cohen, 2003; Litz, 2003; Omer & Schnyder, 2003). Addressing this requires additional knowledge about children's vulnerability to trauma-related disorders, and in particular, what clusters of pre-event, event-related, and post-event variables will predict subsequent impaired functioning (e.g., Yehuda, McFarlane, & Shalev, 1998). The data reported above suggest the importance of assessing key aspects of children's involvement in incidents of IPV, in conjunction with prior risk factors such as trauma history. From a clinical perspective, the value of a police-mental health partnership such as CDPP lies in its ability to (a) provide psycho-education (including safety planning) for families, (b) screen children for traumatic exposure and functioning, and (c) broker services for children who (due to the severity of their exposure, pre-existing risk factors, or a combination thereof) may subsequently benefit from clinical intervention. This type of intervention is consistent with a growing body of literature that documents the need for effective interventions for children exposed to violence to be community-based and multi-systemic (Fantuzzo et al., 1997; Geffner et al., 2000; Groves & Gewirtz, 2006; Kerig, 2003). Though challenging, attempts to count the "hard-to-count" and measure the "hard-to-measure" provide a critical basis for improving the standard of care for children exposed to IPV.

NOTES

1. For example, in Hennepin County, Minnesota, county child protection policies mandate reporting of IPV incidents in which children were present in the home and (a) were directly involved in the violence (e.g., by calling 911); or (b) where the incident involved a weapon or was charged as a felony case. Police report all cases meeting these criteria to child protection.

2. The CDPP team attempted to contact all families at least one time, within a week of the violent event. When families were out, and did not contact the team or return phone calls, the case "timed out," and no more attempts were made to contact the family with regard to this incident. Approximately 90% families were offered services. During the time period from which data were gathered, services were available three nights per week. Currently, however, services are available throughout Minneapolis 24 hours per day, 7 days per week. (For more information on the program, see Gewirtz et al., 2006.)

3. All police reports are written by the patrol officers first responding to the scene (rather than by the officer accompanying the clinician and advocate). Training by family violence professionals, mental health professionals, and police supervisors was provided to police officers to increase their awareness of the importance of documenting the presence of children on the scene of IPV incidents.

4. Only 61/66 child records had notations of when the CDPP visit occurred (i.e., number of days following the incident), and therefore five records were excluded from the regression.

REFERENCES

Bachman, R., & Coker, A. L. (1995). Police involvement in domestic violence: The interactive effects of victim injury, offender's history of violence, and race. *Violence and Victims, 10*(2), 91–106.

Berkowitz, S. J. (2003). Children exposed to community violence: The rationale for early intervention. *Clinical Child and Family Psychology Review, 6*(4), 293–302.

Chamberlain, L. (2008). Ten lessons learned in Alaska: Home visitation and intimate partner violence. *Journal of Emotional Abuse, 8*(1/2), 205–216.

Cicchetti, D., & Toth, S. (1995). A developmental psychopathology perspective on child abuse and neglect. *Journal of the American Academy of Child and Adolescent Psychiatry, 34*(5), 541–565.

Cohen, J. A. (2003). Treating acute posttraumatic reactions in children and adolescents. *Biological Psychiatry, 53*, 827–833.

Edleson, J. L. (1999). Children's witnessing of adult domestic violence. *Journal of Interpersonal Violence, 14*(8), 839–870.

Edleson, J. L., Mbilinyi, L. F., Beeman, S. K., & Hagemeister, A. K. (2003). How children are involved in adult domestic violence: results from a four-city telephone survey. *Journal of Interpersonal Violence, 18*(1), 18–32.

Ernst, A. A., Weiss, S. J., & Enright-Smith, S. (2006). Child witnesses and victims in homes with adult intimate partner violence. *Academy of Emergency Medicine, 13*(6), 696–699.

Fantuzzo, J., Boruch, R., Beriama, A., Atkins, M., & Marcus, S. (1997). Domestic violence and children: prevalence and risk in five major US cities. *Journal of the American Academy of Child and Adolescent Psychiatry, 36*(1), 116–122.

Geffner, R., Jaffe, P., & Sudermann, M. (2000). *Children exposed to domestic violence: Current issues in research, intervention, prevention, and policy development.* Binghampton, NY: Haworth Press.

Gewirtz, A., & Edleson, J. L. (2007). Young children's exposure to intimate partner violence: Towards a developmental risk and resilience framework for research and intervention. *Journal of Family Violence, 22*(3), 151–163.

Gewirtz, A., Harris, D., & Avendano, M. J. (2006). Improving access to care for traumatized children: Law enforcement-mental health collaborations for child witnesses to violence. *CURA Reporter, 36*(2), 28–34.

Gewirtz, A., Miller, H., Weidner, R., & Zehm, K. (2006). Domestic violence cases involving children: effects of an evidence-based prosecution approach. *Violence and Victims, 21*(2), 213–229.

Green, B., Korol, M., & Grace, M. (1991). Children and disaster: Age, gender and parental effects on PTSD symptoms. *Journal of the American Academy of Child and Adolescent Psychiatry, 30*, 945–951.

Groves, B., & Gewirtz, A. (2006). Interventions and promising approaches for children exposed to domestic violence. In M. Feerick & G. Silverman (Eds.), *Children exposed to domestic violence* (pp. 106–136). Baltimore, MD: Brookes Publishing.

Groves, B. M. (2003). *Children who see too much: Lessons from the child witness to violence project.* Boston, MA: Houghton Mifflin.

Jaffe, P., Wolfe, D., & Wilson, S. (1990). *Children of battered women.* Newbury Park, CA: Sage.

Jouriles, E. N., McDonald, R., Stephens, N., Norwood, W., Spiller, L. C., & Ware, H. S. (1998). Breaking the cycle of violence: Helping families departing from battered women's shelters. In G. W. Holden, R. A. Geffner & E. N. Jouriles (Eds.), *Children exposed to marital violence: Theory, research, and applied issues* (pp. 337–370). Washington, DC: American Psychological Association.

Kerig, P. K. (2003). In search of protective processes for children exposed to violence. In R. Geffner, R. S. Igelman, & J. Zellner (Eds.), *The effects of intimate partner violence on children* (pp. 149–181). Binghamton, NY: Haworth Press.

Kracke, K., & Cohen, E. (2008). The Safe Start Initiative: Building and disseminating knowledge to support children exposed to violence. *Journal of Emotional Abuse, 8*(1/2), 155–174.

Kracke, K., & Hahn, H. (2008). The nature and extent of childhood exposure to violence: What we know, why we don't know more, and why it matters. *Journal of Emotional Abuse, 8*(1/2), 29–49.

La Greca, A., Silverman, W., Vernberg, E., & Prinstein, M. (1996). Symptoms of post-traumatic stress in children after Hurricane Andrew: A prospective study. *Journal of Consulting and Clinical Psychology, 64*(4), 712–723.

Litz, B. T. (2003). *Early intervention for trauma and traumatic loss.* New York: Guilford Press.

Marans, S., & Adelman, A. (1997). Experiencing violence in a developmental context. In J. D. Osofsky (Ed.), *Children in a violent society* (pp. 202–222). New York: Guilford Press.

Margolin, G., & Gordis, E. B. (2000). The effects of family and community violence on children. *Annual Review of Psychology, 51,* 445–479.

McCloskey, L. A., Figueredo, A. J., & Koss, M. P. (1995). The effects of systemic family violence on children's mental health. *Child Development, 66*(5), 1239–1261.

McCloskey, L. A., & Walker, M. (2000). Posttraumatic stress in children exposed to family violence and single-event trauma. *Journal of the American Academy of Child and Adolescent Psychiatry, 39*(1), 108–115.

McMahon, S., Grant, K., Compas, B., Thurm, A., & Ey, S. (2003). Stress and psychopathology in children and adolescents: is there evidence of specificity? *Journal of Child Psychology and Psychiatry, 44*(1), 107.

Mihalic, S. W., & Elliott, D. (1997). If violence is domestic, does it really count? *Journal of Family Violence, 12*(3), 293–311.

Nader, K., Pynoos, R., Fairbanks, L., & Frederick, C. (1990). Children's PTSD reactions one year after a sniper attack at their school. *American Journal of Psychiatry, 147*(11), 1526–1530.

O'Brien, M., John, R. S., Margolin, G., & Erel, O. (1994). Reliability and diagnostic efficacy of parents' reports regarding children's exposure to marital aggression. *Violence and Victims, 9,* 45–62.

Omer, R., & Schnyder, U. E. (2003). *Reconstructing early intervention after trauma: Innovations in the care of survivors.* Oxford: Oxford University Press.

Osofsky, J. D. (1997). *Children in a violent society.* New York: Guilford Press.

Osofsky, J. D. (2003). Prevalence of children's exposure to domestic violence and child maltreatment: Implications for prevention and intervention. *Clinical Child and Family Psychology Review, 6*(3), 161–170.

Pine, D. S., & Cohen, J. A. (2002). Trauma in children and adolescents: risk and treatment of psychiatric sequelae. *Biological Psychiatry, 51*(7), 519–531.

Pynoos, R. S., & Nader, K. (1989). Children's memory and proximity to violence. *Journal of the American Academy of Child and Adolescent Psychiatry, 28*(2), 236–241.

Rosenbaum, A., & O'Leary, K. D. (1981). Children: The unintended victims of marital violence. *American Journal of Orthopsychiatry, 51*(4), 692–699.

Schaffer, D., Gould, M. S., Brasic, J., Ambrosini, P., Fisher, P., Bird, H., et al. (1983). A children's global assessment scale (CGAS). *Archives of General Psychiatry, 40,* 1228–1231.

Straus, M., & Gelles, R. (1990). *Physical violence in American families.* New Brunswick, NJ: Transaction Books.

Yehuda, R., McFarlane, A. C., & Shalev, A. Y. (1998). Predicting the development of posttraumatic stress disorder from the acute response to a traumatic event. *Biological Psychiatry, 44*(12), 1305–1313.

Zuckerman, B., Augustyn, M., Groves, B. M., & Parker, S. (1995). Silent victims revisited: the special case of domestic violence. *Pediatrics, 96*(3 Pt 1), 511–513.

The Physiological and Traumatic Effects of Childhood Exposure to Intimate Partner Violence

Steve Stride
Robert Geffner
Alan Lincoln

Exposure to intimate partner violence (IPV) or abuse may be considered a form of psychological abuse that can produce traumatic stress. However, there is debate in the legal arena whether exposure to IPV alone, without other forms of abuse, is child maltreatment. Nevertheless, 3–4 million American households experience IPV every year (Kessman, 2000). Jaffe, Wolfe, and Wilson (1990) reviewed studies examining the rates of IPV exposure for children and estimated that 68–80% of children in homes where IPV has occurred are exposed to and likely affected by it (see Kracke & Hahn, 2008, this issue, for a discussion on definitions of abuse as well as the incidence and prevalence of childhood exposure to violence (CEV)).

Research during the past 15 years has established that exposure to IPV is a major risk factor for post-traumatic stress disorder (PTSD) in children (Arroyo & Eth, 1995; Jaffe, Suderman, & Reitzel, 1992; Kerig, Fedorowicz, Brown, & Warren, 2000). Unresolved, severe, and repeated trauma can result in a series of negative events (e.g., Perry, Pollard, Blakely, Baker, & Vigilante, 1995), including severe psychological and physiological impairments for the child. Specifically, traumatized children who experience increased stress may experience a stress response and physiological changes resulting from the trauma.

TRAUMA, PTSD, AND THE STRESS RESPONSE

Post-traumatic stress disorder involves an increased sensitivity to stressful cues and bodily responses, such as abnormally high heart rates, avoidance of situations that cause stress, and re-experiencing stressful events as if they are occurring in the present (American Psychiatric Association

[APA], 2000). Kitzmann, Gaylord, Holt, and Kenny (2003), Graham-Berman and Levendosky (1998), Landis (1989), Lehman (1997), and Logan and Graham-Berman (1999) found that children exposed to their father assaulting their mother had high levels of trauma symptoms, post-traumatic stress, and anxiety. In fact, both Landis and Lehman found that over half of the children in their samples showed symptoms of PTSD.

THE PHYSIOLOGICAL AND NEURODEVELOPMENTAL EFFECTS OF CHILDHOOD EXPOSURE TO IPV

While the relationship between stress and trauma and their resulting physiological reactions has been well documented, more research is being conducted with respect to their neurodevelopmental and neuropsychological aspects. Perry et al. (1995) hypothesized that traumatic experience, such as childhood exposure to IPV, results in sensitization of neurons, with subsequent minor stressors potentially resulting in a full-blown stress response. This stress response keeps a child safe by making him/her more aware and alert of surroundings. However, when there is no future threat, the memory of a past traumatic experience may work against the child. The fixated memory may negatively affect the perception and interpretation of future events. These stressful memories may have an immediate impact on the neurodevelopment of the child and appear to have implications in adulthood.

Variance in the activity of neurons depends on the pattern, intensity, and frequency of neural activity. When the pattern of neural activation is more intense and frequent, the internal representation that results is more permanent. Perry et al. (1995) refer to this representation as the processing template that results from experiences and through which all future information is filtered. The more frequently the neurons are activated, the greater the internalization of information (LeDoux, Iwata, & Cicchetti, 1988).

Stress also impacts our neurochemical system. Cortisol is a hormone that is part of the parasympathetic response to stress and slows down the body during and after removal of a stressor (Rivier & Plotsky, 1986). Lovallo and Thomas (2000) found that during episodes of fear-related stress, high levels of cortisol are pumped into the bloodstream (Lovallo, Pincomb, Brackett, & Wilson, 1990). The level of cortisol increases as the duration and intensity of the stressor increases. For example, Nejtek (2002) discovered that there is a difference in emotional stress perceptions and salivary cortisol response based on intensity of emotional events. Participants exposed to a high stress paradigm exhibited more emotional stress and had higher salivary cortisol levels (1.05 to 1.17 micrograms [ug]/deciliter [dL]) than those exposed to a low stress paradigm (1.05 to .99ug/dL). Cortisol rose from baseline during high stress paradigm and dropped after removal of the stressor. This supports the view that acute stress leads to release of cortisol. When the intensity of the stressor is high, the cortisol level is high (Seyle, 1976).

The purpose for increased cortisol production is to calm the body down during the stressor and keep the individual calm after removal of the stressor (Uchino, Cacioppo, Malarkey, & Glaser, 1995). After removal of the stressor or threat, cortisol acts on the hippocampus, amygdala, and the hypothalamic-pituitary-adrenal (HPA) axis through negative feedback inhibition (DeKloet & Reul, 1987) until basal hormone level is restored (McEwen, DeKloet, & Rostene, 1987). Some studies indicate that PTSD patients have suppressed cortisol levels (Yehuda, Giller, Southwick, Lowy, & Mason, 1991). However, a recent study by Lindley, Carlson, and Benoit (2004) showed that PTSD patients had higher concentrations of cortisol than the comparison group. Overall, PTSD has been associated with higher concentrations of cortisol.

Additional studies have focused on the process by which these physiological changes occur. The amygdala simultaneously projects to the solitary tract to stimulate parasympathetic responses (Kapp, Pascoe, & Bixler, 1984). The central amygdala projects to the bed nucleus of the stria terminalis to initiate the HPA axis response (Roozendaal, Koolhaas, & Bohus, 1992). The parasympathetic response helps to constrain the sympathetic discharge by activating the HPA axis. Brain neuropeptides stimulate the hypothalamus to release corticotropin-releasing factors. Other regulatory neuropeptides stimulate the pituitary release of adrenocorticotropic hormone and stimulate the adrenal gland to produce cortisol (King, Mandansky, King, Fletcher, & Brewer, 2001). Individuals with PTSD may have alterations in the sympathetic and parasympathetic nervous systems that may have an impact on responsiveness to threatening and nonthreatening stimuli. This means that they frequently have overactive sympathetic and parasympathetic responses. The impact of these physiological changes may result in symptoms of PTSD, and have been evident in trauma survivors (Buckley & Kaloupek, 2001).

There is increased sympathetic nervous system activation and a high level of catecholamines under basal (Yehuda, Resnick, Schmeidler, Yang, & Pitman, 1998a) and stimulated conditions (McFall, Murburg, & Ko,

1990). Catecholamines provide energy to vital organs and mobilize the body for action in response to a stressor. Individuals with PTSD are over-reactive when a stressor is presented and are prepared for action even when there is no threat. When presented with a stressful stimulus, they have exhibited higher heart rates than those in a comparison group (Brownley, Hurwitz, & Schneiderman, 2000). Another study with over 2500 participants revealed higher resting heart rates in participants with PTSD than in trauma-exposed individuals without PTSD and nontrauma exposed individuals (Buckley & Kaloupek, 2001).

Muraoka, Carlson, and Chemtob (1998) compared resting heart rates among 11 Vietnam veterans with combat experience and PTSD to 7 noncombat veterans with no PTSD. While the results of the study should be interpreted cautiously due to the small sample size, they supported the position that individuals with PTSD have higher heart rate levels. Post-traumatic stress disorder patients also tend to have a higher heart rate across different settings (Beckham et al., 2000; Gerardi, Keane, Cahoon, & Klauminzer, 1994; Orr, Meyeroff, Edwards, & Pitman, 1998).

Individuals exposed to IPV as children often exhibit signs of PTSD in adulthood if there has been no intervention. The literature has indicated that PTSD patients tend to have increased heart rates in general and produce higher amounts of cortisol. The purpose of the present study was to examine whether individuals exposed to IPV as children differed from individuals who experienced physical/sexual abuse as children or individuals with no child-hood abuse history in the following: (a) heart rate during a stress condition; (b) cortisol levels during a stress condition; and (c) trauma symptoms.

METHODS

Participants

Participants were recruited from psychology classes at a Southern California college. One hundred thirty-three participants were contacted and screened for inclusion in the study. Participants were eligible if they were not pregnant; not using oral contraceptives; had similar nighttime sleep cycles (going to bed between 10:00 P.M. and midnight, and awaking between 6:00 A.M. and 9:00 A.M.); did not smoke; weighed less than 200 pounds; and were willing to consent to participate in research lasting approximately 2 hours. These criteria were established in order to control for factors that could influence cortisol levels according to extant research. Potential participants with a history of heart problems were also excluded due to the risk of heart trauma during the stressor. Forty-three potential participants were excluded based on the above criteria, resulting in a sample of 90 students. Eight participants (three in the exposure group, two in the physical/sexual abuse group, and three in the nonabuse group) did not show up for their appointment. Thus, the final sample consisted of 82 participants. Power analyses determined that the group size was sufficient for the planned analyses.

The 82 participants ranged in age from 18–30 and included 24 males and 58 females. The participant pool consisted of 1 Native American (1.2%), 10 Asians (12.2%), 20 African Americans (24.4%), 37 Hispanics (45.1%), 13 Caucasians (15.9%), and 1 of other racial/ethnic identity (1.2%). Groups were identified based on self-reported history of physical/sexual abuse, exposure to IPV, or no abuse. The groups included 31 participants in the exposure group (those exposed to IPV as children but not physically or sexually abused), 22 in the physical/sexual abuse group (those directly abused as children), and 29 participants in the nonabuse group (those with no history of abuse or exposure).

Procedures

Participants were asked if they would like to participate in a study involving stress response. They were given 10 points of extra credit in their psychology class if they completed the entire protocol. Potential participants were screened for eligibility, and those who were eligible then completed informed consent procedures. Following completion of the experimental protocol (described later), all participants were debriefed and provided with a list of treatment resources that were available. Referral arrangements to free counseling services were also made available because of the potential discomfort of the stressor. All study procedures were reviewed and approved by the Institutional Review Board at Alliant International University, San Diego.

Experimental Protocol

At baseline, participants' heart rate was measured and they were given a salivary cortisol test while listening to and participating in relaxation exercises. They then watched a 5-minute video (the stressor) that showed a child witnessing IPV, and heart rate and salivary cortisol were again measured. A relaxation phase followed the stressor, during which salivary cortisol was measured once and heart rate was measured four times.

Measures

Heart Rate

Heart rate was measured using an electrocardiogram (ECG) (Hewlett Packard M1094A, Palo Alto, CA). Heart rate was measured in number of heart beats per minute (bpm). Average resting heart rate is usually between 60–80 bpm (Brownley et al., 2000).

Salivary Cortisol

Salivary cortisol was measured using the Salimetrics HS-Cortisol High Sensitivity Salivary Cortisol Enzyme Immunoassay Kit (Salimetrics LLC, State College, PA), which was designed for the quantitative in-vitro diagnostic measurement of salivary cortisol. Salimetrics verified the precision of the salivary cortisol test by examining seven saliva samples containing different levels of endogenous cortisol. Samples were spiked with known quantities of cortisol and assayed.

PTSD

The detailed assessment of post-traumatic stress (DAPS; Briere, 2001) is an objective measure of trauma exposure and a post-traumatic response inventory. It contains 104 statements with five response categories ranging from *"in the last day"* to *"a year ago or longer."* The DAPS has two validity scales and 11 clinical scales. These scales evaluate a range of trauma-relevant parameters, including lifetime exposure to traumatic events; immediate cognitive, emotional, and dissociative responses to a specified trauma; the symptoms of PTSD and Acute Stress Disorder (ASD) as defined by the *Diagnostic and Statistical Manual of Mental Disorders* (APA, 2000); the likelihood of a PTSD or ASD diagnosis; and three associated features of PTSD (post-traumatic dissociation, suicidal thoughts, and substance abuse). The post-traumatic stress total scale is a summary score used in the present study to evaluate overall level of PTSD symptoms (intrusive re-experiencing, avoidance/numbing, and autonomic hyperarousal). The Peritraumatic Dissociation Scale was also used in the analyses. Higher scores on the DAPS scales indicate greater endorsement of PTSD symptoms. The reliability and validity data are available in Briere (2001).

Statistical Analysis

Differences in heart rate and cortisol levels were analyzed using a 3 (abuse type: exposure to IPV, physical/sexual abuse, or no abuse) × 3 (study phase: baseline, stressor, recovery) repeated measures ANOVA. For each of these analyses, Roy's largest root was used to analyze main effects. For the heart rate analysis, recovery was a transformed variable that consisted of the arithmetic mean of the four heart rate measurements obtained during the relaxation phase. Differences between the three groups in PTSD symptoms were analyzed using a one-way ANOVA. For all three outcome measures, pairwise comparisons were conducted to examine differences between individual abuse types and/or between study phases.

RESULTS

Heart Rate

Results of the analyses of heart rate are presented in Table 1. There was a significant abuse type × study phase interaction, $F(2, 29) = 3.17, p < .05$, such that participants who had a history of exposure to IPV had higher heart rates overall ($M = 89.4, SD = 20.2$) and throughout each study phase when compared to the physical/sexual abuse ($M = 83.7, SD = 12.8$) and no abuse group ($M = 80.1, SD = 12.9$). There was also a main effect for study phase ($p = .001$). Examination of the pairwise comparisons for study phase showed that heart rates significantly decreased from the stressor ($M = 86.5, SD = 18.6$) to recovery ($M = 81.4, SD = 15.3; p = .002$), and from baseline ($M = 83.8, SD = 12.9$) to recovery ($M = 81.4, SD = 15.3; p = .009$). Heart rates significantly increased from baseline to stressor ($p = .008$).

Two t tests were conducted to assess differences between the abuse groups during the stressor phase. There was a significant difference between the exposure to IPV group ($M = 96.5, SD = 18.5, t(58) = 3.1, p = 003$) and the no abuse group ($M = 80.3, SD = 11.5$) on heart rate during the stressor. There were no other significant differences in heart rate during the stressor based on group.

Cortisol

Results of the analyses of cortisol levels are presented in Table 2. There was a significant Abuse type × Study Phase interaction, $F(2, 79) = 3.17, p = .047$, such that participants who had a history of IPV exposure ($M = .23, SD = .02$) and physical/sexual abuse ($M = .26, SD = .04$) had higher cortisol levels overall and throughout each study phase when

TABLE 1. Effects of type of abuse and study phase on heart rate

Source	REPEATED MEASURES ANOVA		
	df	F	p
Abuse type	2,79	1.54	.22
Study phase	2,78	14.70***	.001
Abuse type × study phase	2,79	3.40*	.04

Source	PAIRWISE COMPARISONS		
	Mean Difference	t (df)	P
Baseline – stressor	2.66	2.72(2, 79)	.008
Stressor – recovery	−5.16**	3.59(2, 79)	.002
Baseline – recovery	−2.51**	2.67(2, 79)	.009
IPV exposed – no abuse	8.73**	3.33(2, 58)	.01
IPV exposed – phys/sex abuse	4.59	1.59(2, 51)	.205
Phys/sex abuse – No abuse	4.15	1.64(2, 49)	.258

Source	MEANS AND STANDARD DEVIATIONS		
	Baseline (M, SD)	Stressor (M, SD)	Recovery (M, SD)
IPV exposed	87.4, 14.5	96.5, 18.5	84.3, 17.3
Phy/sex abuse	84.4, 11.4	85.5, 14.3	81.2, 12.7
No abuse	80.6, 14.5	80.3, 11.5	79.3, 12.6

*p < .05; **p < .01; ***p < .001.

compared to the no abuse group ($M = .19$, $SD = .02$). There was also a main effect for study phase, $F(2, 78) = 7.86$, $p = .001$, with cortisol levels decreasing for all groups in the study when the stressor was presented. Examination of the pairwise comparisons showed that cortisol levels significantly decreased from baseline ($M = .28$, $SD = .02$) to the stressor phase ($M = .24$, $SD = .01$; $p < .001$), from the stressor phase ($M = .24$, $SD = .01$) to the recovery phase ($M = .21$, $SD = .09$; $p = .001$), and from baseline ($M = .28$, $SD = .20$) to the recovery phase ($M = .21$, $SD = .09$; $p < .001$).

Two t tests were conducted to assess differences between the groups during the stressor. Those with a physical/sexual abuse history ($M = .27$, $SD = .06$; $t(2, 49) = 2.34$, $p = .02$) had significantly higher cortisol levels during the stressor compared to nonabused participants ($M = .18$, $SD = .02$). The IPV exposure group did not significantly differ from the no abuse group in cortisol levels during the stressor. Thus, individuals who

TABLE 2. Effects of type of abuse and study phase on cortisol

Source	REPEATED MEASURES ANOVA		
	df	F	p
Abuse Type	2,79	3.46*	.036
Study phase	2,78	7.86***	.001
Abuse type × study phase	2,79	3.17*	.047

Source	PAIRWISE COMPARISONS		
	Mean Difference	t(df)	P
Baseline – stressor	−.07ug/dl***	3.72(2, 79)	.001
Stressor – recovery	−.04ug/dl***	3.28(2, 79)	.001
Baseline – recovery	−.11ug/dl***	4.02(2, 79)	.001
IPV exposed – no abuse	.04ug/dl	1.03(2, 58)	.17
IPV exposed – phys/sex abuse	−.03ug/dl	.44(2, 51)	.73
Phys/sex abuse – no abuse	.07ug/dl	1.76(2, 49)	.11

Source	MEANS AND STANDARD DEVIATIONS		
	Baseline (M, SD)	Stressor (M, SD)	Recovery (M, SD)
IPV exposed	.27, .03	.24, .02	.17, .01
Phy/sex abuse	.32, .05	.27, .06	.20, .03
No abuse	.23, .02	.18, .02	.15, .01

*$p < .05$; **$p < .1$; ***$p < .001$.

had a history of physical/sexual abuse appeared to have higher stress levels than nonabused populations when a stressor was presented as indicated by the higher cortisol level. However, those who were exposed to IPV did not differ from nonabused participants in their cortisol levels during the stressor.

PTSD Symptoms

There were significant differences in PTSD symptoms by abuse type, $F(2, 79) = 18.65$, $p = .036$. Pairwise comparisons indicated that those who experienced physical/sexual abuse or who were exposed to IPV had higher levels of post-traumatic stress than those with no abuse history ($p < .001$ for both analyses; see Table 3). IPV-exposed and physically and/or sexually abused participants did not significantly differ in reported levels of post-traumatic stress.

TABLE 3. Effects of abuse type on DAPS scores

Source	ANOVA		
	df	F	p
Abuse Type	2,79	18.65***	.036

Source	PAIRWISE COMPARISONS		
	Mean Difference	t(df)	p
IPV exposed – no abuse	20.08***	3.70(2, 58)	.001
IPV exposed – phys/sex abuse	0.08	0.02(2, 51)	.98
Phys/sex abuse – no abuse	20.00***	4.05(2, 49)	.001

Source	MEANS AND STANDARD DEVIATIONS		
	(M, SD)		
IPV exposed	66.5, 22.4		
Phy/sex abuse	66.4, 19.7		
No abuse	46.4, 8.4		

$*p < .05; **p < .1; ***p < .001.$

Pairwise comparisons indicated that those who experienced physical/sexual abuse ($M = 67.0$, $SD = 11.3$; $t(2, 49) = 4.58$, $p = .001$) and those exposed to IPV ($M = 64.0$, $SD = 14.1$; $t(2, 58) = 3.56$, $p = .001$) had higher peritraumatic dissociation scores on the DAPS than those with no abuse history ($M = 52.0$, $SD = 11.7$). IPV-exposed and physically and/or sexually abused participants did not significantly differ in peritraumatic dissociation scores.

DISCUSSION

While exposure to IPV has been shown to be a major risk factor for PTSD in children (Arroyo & Eth, 1995), studies have not examined the long-term physiological effects of such exposure. The present study examined whether the symptoms of those exposed to IPV mimicked those seen in studies of trauma survivors with PTSD. Post-traumatic stress disorder patients described in the literature have higher resting heart rates than trauma-exposed individuals without PTSD and nontrauma exposed individuals (Buckley & Kaloupek, 2001). Similarly, in the present study those exposed to IPV group had higher resting heart rates than those who had been physically or sexually abused and those who had no abuse history. This may mean that participants who were exposed to IPV over a long period of time experience as much or more chronic stress than physically or sexually abused participants, and are similar to PTSD patients as defined in the literature.

Participants with physical/sexual abuse histories had the highest cortisol levels and diagnosable trauma symptoms for PTSD. This may indicate that abuse which has a physical component triggers the physiological stress response of cortisol increase more intensely compared to other categories of abuse. This explanation makes sense because PTSD patients experience higher levels of stress than comparison groups. It is thus expected that cortisol levels would also be higher in this population because more is needed to bring PTSD patients back to homeostasis. If this is true, then PTSD patients and individuals who have been physically or sexually abused may actually be similar in cortisol output. It is clear from this study that those who have experienced or been exposed to violence endure a great deal of stress. It is reasonable to assume that these individuals also need high volumes of cortisol to return to homeostasis. A possible explanation for the nonsignificant cortisol level in the exposure to IPV group may be related to dissociation during the stressor. The video stressor used in the present study depicted an IPV scene, and may have caused the exposure to IPV group to dissociate more than the other groups during the video. Overall, those exposed to IPV and those who had been physically or sexually abused reported significantly higher peritraumatic dissociation scores than those in the no abuse group. Since both of these abuse groups tend to dissociate under stress, one hypothesis for the lower cortisol levels in the exposure to IPV group is that these subjects dissociated more during the stressor than did those who had a history of physical/ sexual abuse. That is not surprising in retrospect since the stressor was directly related and likely similar to their childhood experiences, which could have produced a more traumatic response that then triggered the dissociation defenses. The increased heart rates obtained in the exposure to IPV group substantiated that they were under stress, and in fact their heart rates were even higher than the physical/sexual abuse group. Thus, it makes sense that dissociation would be triggered if they have a tendency toward this as a coping mechanism. Since dissociation has a numbing effect after the sympathetic response has taken place, this would then lower the cortisol levels (as was found). In other words, dissociation actually accentuates the parasympathetic response. Less cortisol is necessary to bring the individual back to homeostasis in abuse/exposure groups if the participants dissociate during stressors to avoid the emotional trauma.

Overall, there were conflicting results when comparing the IPV exposure group and the physical or sexual abuse group regarding the physiological symptoms of trauma. The expectation is that an individual who has a trauma history would have higher heart rate and cortisol levels when exposed to stressful conditions as compared with a no abuse group. The expected result for higher heart rate overall and during stressful conditions held true when the exposure to IPV group was compared to the no abuse group. However, the physical or sexual abuse group did not have a significantly higher heart rate than the no abuse group. Further, the expected results for higher cortisol levels among individuals with trauma histories when compared to those with no abuse histories held true for the physical or sexual abuse group during the stressor. However, the expectation that cortisol level would be significantly higher overall and during the stressor for the IPV exposure group when compared to the no abuse group was not supported.

Some of the present results concur with the findings of Lindley et al. (2004), in which PTSD patients with a history of trauma actually produced higher concentrations of cortisol. A possible explanation for the differences in cortisol level may have to do with differences in the populations. In the studies where consistently lower cortisol levels were found, the participants were not diagnosed with PTSD and the nature of the trauma was acute. For instance, Yehuda et al. (1998a) measured cortisol levels in subjects who had been raped and found low cortisol levels. This suggests that those with pervasive trauma histories, such as physical or sexual abuse or IPV exposure, may experience more overall chronic stress than individuals with acute trauma or no trauma history. This is evidenced by significantly higher heart rates overall and during stressors as well as PTSD symptoms that reached clinical levels. The system that produces cortisol is thus highly active in trauma victims, which helps them deal with the increased level of stress. The present results indicate that there are similarities in cortisol production for physically or sexually abused participants in this study and some PTSD patients described in the literature.

Implications

The present results demonstrate the need for early intervention for children who are living in homes with IPV. Even though children were not a part of this study, the results showed the long-term impact of childhood exposure to IPV on adults. Trauma symptoms may be decreased or eliminated if a child exposed to IPV is treated quickly. Timely intervention may curtail the long-term symptom of increased heart rate during stress.

As found in this study, stressors had a significant impact on those exposed to IPV. This presents another risk factor because individuals with high heart rates are vulnerable to heart disease (Cloitre, Cohen, Edelman, & Han, 2001). Therefore, identifying adults who were exposed to IPV may help in the early identification of people at higher risk for heart and blood pressure problems, even if they may not be aware of their risks. Since the findings of the present study also showed a decrease in the heart rate after relaxation, this also has treatment implications, and offers a way to help those with such stress reactions.

Another important implication concerns the way children learn to cope with the trauma of IPV exposure. In the present study, those in both the IPV exposure as well as the physical/sexual abuse groups tended to dissociate as a coping mechanism. This may occur whenever they are under stress, and may not be a healthy way of coping as adults. Identifying children and adolescents who dissociate under stress may also help in initiating referrals at earlier ages for trauma therapy so that the effects do not continue into adulthood.

Limitations

This study was conducted on a nonclinical population of college students who had not been to therapy. A clinical sample would have had distinctly defined diagnoses that could have been tested, and the differences between them might have shown up more clearly. In addition, one mediator of cortisol response that was not controlled in the present study was alcohol use. Chronic consumption of alcohol is associated with increased cortisol production (Badrick et al., 2008). This confound may be a concern, since it is possible that both the exposure to the IPV group and the physical/sexual abuse group were higher than the no abuse group because of chronic alcohol consumption. Finally, the video stressor used in the present study depicted an IPV scene, and may have affected the physiological and post-traumatic symptom results. A different scenario may have produced somewhat different results. Indeed, there was no prior research demonstrating that the scene actually produced stress. However, it was assumed that the video caused stress due to the heart rate increases.

FUTURE RESEARCH

Future study should further examine heart rates of individuals who have been exposed to IPV. Post-traumatic stress disorder patients described in the literature have elevated heart rates during sleep (Muraoka et al., 1998) and across different situations (Beckham et al., 2000). Studying the heart rate of individuals exposed to IPV during sleep and in different situations would be important in gaining a clearer understanding of how the heart and person responds. A direct comparison under these conditions should be made between PTSD patients without an abuse history and individuals exposed to IPV in order to show the specific similarities or differences between these two populations. Future research should also include a control group without a stressor, and compare them to those who had a stressor. This design would then show more definitively if the stressor actually had an impact on the participants. Introducing different types of stressors would also be helpful in understanding how they impact different trauma populations. Finally, it is suggested that heart rate be measured on an average over the time intervals. The use of computer software in measuring heart rate or other physiological responses is recommended as it has the capacity to record ongoing heart rate throughout the protocol, which would allow the researcher to control for and analyze abnormal fluctuations in heart rate and would enhance the reliability of the data.

Future studies need to examine the neurochemistry of the stress response in individuals who have been exposed to IPV. There is still not a clear understanding of neurochemistry within the population of adults who have been exposed to IPV. These studies should provide information about potential psychopharmacological options available for trauma symptoms. More studies on the neurochemistry of cortisol may allow for the development of medications that would mimic its effect on receptor sites. This could bring relief from stress symptoms to individuals with PTSD, individuals who have been exposed to IPV, and individuals who have been physically or sexually abused.

Use of the Suicidality Supplementary Scale on the DAPS along with another depression measure should be considered in future research, along with a clinically depressed comparison group, as the results of this study showed that the physically or sexually abused group had high cortisol levels. Individuals with increased cortisol are prone to developing depression (Yehuda, Siever, & Teicher, 1998b). A comparison group would allow researchers to see whether an IPV exposure group or a physically or sexually abused group has similar physiological and psychological symptoms when compared to a clinically depressed group.

CONCLUSION

The results of the present study showed that adults who were exposed to IPV as children experienced long-term physiological changes, including high resting heart rates, slightly high cortisol levels, and significant trauma symptoms. These results show that exposure to IPV may have a long-term impact on adult sensitivity to post-traumatic stress that is similar to the long-term effects of physical and/or sexual abuse. Being aware of the long-term impact of exposure to IPV has implications for policies concerning the manner in which communities react to and deal with IPV cases. Too often, state and community agency policies and procedures, as well as legal statutes, make strong distinctions in reporting, intervention options, and handling of exposure to IPV cases in comparison to physical or sexual abuse ones. There are usually clear mandates for handling the latter situations, but too often the former are minimized or ignored. The results of the present research indicate the fallacy of this approach, and suggest that those exposed to IPV have many similar traumatic symptoms and effects years later if there has been no intervention. Trauma symptoms may be decreased or eliminated if a child exposed to IPV is treated quickly. Timely intervention may curtail the long-term symptoms of increased heart rate, high cortisol production during a stressor, and high levels of stress.

REFERENCES

American Psychiatric Association (APA) (2000). *Diagnostic and statistical manual of mental disorders* (4th ed.). Washington, DC: Author.

Arroyo, W., & Eth, S. (1995). Assessment following violence-witnessing trauma. In E. Peled, P. G. Jaffe, & J. L. Edelson (Eds.), *Ending the cycle of violence: Community response to children of battered women* (pp. 27–42). Thousand Oaks, CA: Sage.

Badrick, E., Bobak, M., Britton, A., Kirschbaum, C., Marmot, M., & Kumari, M. (2008). The relationship between alcohol consumption and cortisol secretion in an aging cohort. *The Journal of Clinical Endocrinology and Metabolism, 93*(3), 750–757.

Beckham, J. C., Feldman, M. E., Barefoot, J. C., Fairbank, J. A., Helms, M. J., Haney, T. L., et al. (2000). Ambulatory cardiovascular activity in Vietnam combat veterans with and without posttraumatic stress disorder. *Journal of Consulting and Clinical Psychology, 68*(2), 269–276.

Briere, J. (2001). *Detailed assessment of posttraumatic stress (DAPS)*. Odessa, FL: Psychological Assessment Resources.

Brownley, K. A., Hurwitz, B. E., & Schneiderman, N. (2000). Cardiovascular psychophysiology. In J. T. Cacioppo, L. G. Tassinary, & G. G. Bernston, (Eds.), *Handbook of psychophysiology* (2nd ed., pp. 224–264). Cambridge, MA; Cambridge University Press.

Buckley, T. C., & Kaloupek, D. G. (2001). A meta-analytic examination of basal cardiovascular activity in post-traumatic stress disorder. *Psychometric Medicine, 63*(4), 585–594.

Cloitre, M., Cohen, L.R., Edelman, R.E., & Han, H. (2001). Posttraumatic stress disorder and extent of trauma exposure as correlates of medical problems and perceived health among women with childhood abuse. *Women Health, 34(3)*, 1–17.

DeKloet, E. R., & Reul, J. M. (1987). Feedback action and tonic influence of glucocorticoids of brain function: a concept arising from the heterogeneity of brain receptor systems. *Psychoneuroendicronology, 12*, 83–105.

Gerardi, R. J., Keane, T. M., Cahoon, B.J. & Klauminzer, G. W. (1994). An in vivo assessment of physiological arousal in posttraumatic stress disorder. *Journal of Abnormal Psychology, 103*(4), 825–827.

Graham-Berman, S. A., & Levendosky, A. A. (1998). Traumatic stress symptoms in children of battered women. *Journal of Interpersonal Violence, 13*, 111–128.

Jaffe, P. G., Suderman, M., & Reitzel, D. (1992). Child witness of marital violence. In R.T. Ammerman & M. Hersen (Eds.), *Assessment of family violence: A clinical and legal sourcebook* (pp. 313–331). New York: Wiley.

Jaffe, P., Wolfe, D., & Wilson, S. K. (1990). *Children of battered women*. Newbury Park, CA: Sage.

Kapp, B. S., Pascoe, J. P., & Bixler, M. A. (1984). The amygdala: A neuroanatomical systems approach to its contribution to aversive conditioning. In N. Butlers & L. R. Squire (Eds.), *Neuropsychology of memory* (pp. 437–449) New York: Guilford.

Kerig, P. K., Fedorowicz, A. E., Brown, C. A., & Warren, M. (2000). Assessment and intervention for PTSD in children exposed to violence. *Journal of Aggression, Maltreatment & Trauma, 3*(1), 161–184.

Kessmann, J. R. (2000). Domestic violence: Identifying the deadly silence. *Texas Dental Journal, 117*(10), 42–47.

King, J. A., Mandansky, D., King, S., Fletcher, K. E., & Brewer, J. (2001). Early sexual abuse and low cortisol. *Psychiatry and Clinical Neuroscience, 55*(1), 71–74.

Kitzmann, K. M., Gaylord, N. K., Holt, A. R., & Kenny E. D. (2003). Child witnesses to domestic violence: A meta-analytic review. *Journal of Consulting and Clinical Psychology, 71*(2), 339–352.

Kracke, K., & Hahn, H. (2008). The nature and extent of childhood exposure to violence: What we know, why we don't know more, and why it matters. *Journal of Emotional Abuse, 8*(1/2), 29–49.

Landis, T. (1989). *Children in shelters: An exploration of dissociative processes traumatization in some children*. Boulder: University of Colorado.

LeDoux, J.E., Iwata, J., & Cicchetti, P.O. (1988). Different projections of the central amygaloid nucleus mediate autonomic and behavioral correlates of conditioned fear. *Journal of Neuroscience, 8*, 2517–2529.

Lehmann, P. (1997). The development of PTSD in a sample of child witnesses to mother assault. *Journal of Family Violence, 12*(3), 241–257.

Lindley, S. E., Carlson, E. B., & Benoit, M. (2004). Basal and dexamethasone suppressed salivary cortisol concentrations in a community sample of patients with posttraumatic stress disorder. *Biological Psychiatry, 55*(9), 940–945.

Logan, D.E., & Graham-Berman, S.A. (1999). Emotion expression in children exposed to family violence. *Journal of Emotional Abuse, 1(3)*, 39–64.

Lovallo, W. R., Pincomb, G. A., Brackett, D. J., & Wilson, M. F. (1990). Heart rate reactivity as a predictor of neuroendocrine responses to aversive and appetitive challenges. *Psychosomatic Medicine, 52*, 17–26.

Lovallo, W. R., & Thomas, T. L. (2000). Stress hormones in psychophysiological research. In J. T. Cacioppo, L. G. Tassinary, & G. G. Bernston, (Eds.), *Handbook of psychophysiology* (2nd ed., pp. 342–367). Cambridge, MA; Cambridge University Press.

McEwen, B. S., DeKloet, E. R., & Rostene, W. (1987). Adrenal steroid receptors and actions in the nervous system. *Physiology Review, 66*, 1121–1188.

McFall, M., Murburg, M., & Ko, G. (1990). Autonomic response to stress in Vietnam combat veterans with post-traumatic stress disorder. *Biological Psychiatry, 27*, 1165–1175.

Muraoka, M. Y., Carlson, J. G., & Chemtob, C. M. (1998). Twenty-four-hour ambulatory blood pressure and heart rate monitoring in combat-related posttraumatic stress disorder. *Journal of Traumatic Stress, 11*(3), 473–484.

Nejtek, V. A. (2002). High and low emotion events influence emotional stress perceptions and are associated with salivary cortisol response changes in a consecutive stress paradigm. *Psychoneuroendicrinology, 27*(3), 337–352.

Orr, S. P., Meyerhoff, J. L., Edwards, J. V., & Pitman, R. K. (1998). Heart rate and blood pressure resting levels and responses to generic stressors in Vietnam veterans with posttraumatic stress disorder. *Journal of Traumatic Stress, 11*(1), 155–164.

Perry, B. D., Pollard, R. A., Blakely, T. L., Baker, W. L., & Vigilante, D. (1995). Childhood trauma, the neurobiology of adaptation, and "use-dependent" development of the brain: How "states" become "traits." *Infant Mental Health Journal, 16*(4), 271–289.

Rivier, C. L., & Plotsky, C. M. (1986). Mediation by corticotropin releasing factor (CRF) of adenohypophysis hormone secretion. *Annual Review of Physiology, 48*, 475–494.

Roozendaal, B., Koolhaas, J.M., & Bohus, B. (1992). Central amygdaloid involvements in neuroendocrine correlates of conditioned stress response. *Journal of Neuroendocrinology, 4*, 46–52.

Seyle, H. (1976). *The stress of life.* New York: McGraw-Hill.

Uchino, B. N., Cacioppo, J. T., Malarkey, W., & Glaser, R. (1995). Individual differences in cardiac sympathetic control predict endocrine and immune responses to acute psychological stress. *Journal of Personality and Social Psychology, 69*, 736–743.

Yehuda, R., Giller, E. L., Southwick, S. M., Lowy, M. T., & Mason, J. W. (1991). Hypothalamic-pituitary-adrenal dysfunction in posttraumatic stress disorder. *Biological Psychiatry, 30*, 1031–1048.

Yehuda, R., Resnick, H. S., Schmeidler, J., Yang, R. K., & Pitman, R. K. (1998a). Predictors of cortisol and 3-methoxy-4-hydroxyphenlglycol responses in the acute aftermath of rape. *Biological Psychiatry, 43*(11), 855–859.

Yehuda, R., Siever, L., & Teicher, M. H. (1998b). Plasma norepinephrine concentrations and severity of depression in combat PTSD and major depressive disorder. *Biology of Psychiatry, 44*, 56–63.

The Experiences of Adults Exposed to Intimate Partner Violence as Children: An Exploratory Qualitative Study of Resilience and Protective Factors

Staci L. Suzuki
Robert Geffner
Steven F. Bucky

Approximately 3 to 10 million children are exposed to intimate partner violence (IPV) annually (Carlson, 1984; Straus, 1992). According to a recent study, 16–25% of children in two-parent households reported exposure to IPV (Osofsky, 2003). Furthermore, children exposed to IPV usually observe more than one abusive incident between their parents (Straus, 1992).

Studies indicate that the effects of exposure to IPV can lead to emotional, behavioral, social, cognitive, and physical health problems (Fantuzzo & Mohr, 1999; Miller-Perrin & Perrin, 1999; see also Kracke & Hahn, 2008, this issue) both in the short and the long term. Children exposed to IPV often learn abusive behaviors and responses to violence from modeling and watching their parents problem-solve. As a result, many of these children become aggressive and/or passive in their later intimate relationships (Kantor & Jasinski, 1998).

Most research focusing on the short- and long-term effects of childhood maltreatment has investigated the negative pathways and psychopathology associated with development (e.g., Heller, Larrieu, D'Imperio, & Boris, 1999; see also Gewirtz & Medhanie, 2008, this issue). However, these studies have led to "many negative assumptions and deficit-focused models about children growing up under the threat of disadvantage and adversity" (Masten, 2001, p. 227). In contrast, resiliency research investigates the strengths of children exposed to trauma and has since reversed some of the negative hypotheses (Heller et al., 1999; Masten, 2001).

Resiliency and Associated Protective Factors

"The Chinese symbol for the word 'crisis' is a composite of two pictographs: the symbols for 'danger' and 'opportunity'" (Walsh, 1998, p. 7).

Resilience can thus be conceptualized as a process that encapsulates these two symbols. Individuals exposed to trauma overcome adversity in their lives by tapping into their strengths and utilizing effective coping mechanisms (Rutter, 1993). Children who demonstrate the ability to overcome the negative effects associated with exposure to IPV are considered resilient.

Protective factors associated with resilience are assumed to assist with adaptive functioning when facing adversity. Protective factors are those aspects that help to moderate the effects of stress. These factors also have varying definitions. Heller et al. (1999) noted that many researchers view protective factors based on three general principles of the ecological model: "(1) dispositional/temperamental attributes of the child [e.g., responsiveness, independence, intellectual abilities]; (2) a warm and secure family relationship; and (3) the availability of extrafamilial support [e.g., peers, teachers]" (p. 326). The current study identified these areas as internal factors/individual characteristics, family factors, and external factors.

The Current Study

The purpose of the present research was to qualitatively investigate the protective factors that assist in the resiliency process for individuals exposed to IPV as children. In-depth semi-structured interviews with adults exposed to IPV as children provided an understanding into the experiences and perceptions of resilience. By understanding the protective factors in the family that contribute to resilience, clinicians may be better equipped to assist children in overcoming the trauma associated with exposure to IPV.

METHODS

Criteria for Inclusion/Exclusion

The following were the inclusion criteria for this study. Eligible participants had to be adults who: (a) were exposed to IPV in the household in which they were reared; (b) were in nonviolent heterosexual romantic relationships; and (c) had normative mental health, as assessed by the Detailed Assessment of Post-traumatic Stress (DAPS; Briere, 2001) and the Personality Assessment Screener (PAS; Morey, 1997). Adults who were the victims of childhood physical/sexual abuse and those with substance/alcohol abuse problems, as measured by the Michigan Alcoholism Screening Test (MAST; Selzer, 1971) and the Drug Abuse Screening Test (DAST; Skinner, 1982), were excluded.

Participants

Participants were two men and eight women who met the above eligibility criteria. They ranged in age from 23 to 35 years ($M = 29.5$, $SD = 3.8$). Table 1 provides a complete demographic description of the 10 participants.

Measures

Revised Conflict Tactics Scale-Form CA (CTS2-CA)

The CTS2-CA Straus, Hamby, & Warren, 2003 was used to confirm participants' perceptions of exposure to IPV as a child. It is a paper-and-pen measure consisting of 62 items that takes approximately 15 minutes to administer (31 statements assess paternal conflict strategies and 31 items measure maternal conflict strategies). The items are answered on an eight-point Likert scale based on a timeline from "*once that year*" to "*this never happened*." The CTS2-CA consists of four scales. The negotiation scale represents the amount of problem-solving strategies used in intimate relationships, with raw scores ranging from 8 to 120. The psychological aggression scale indicates the amount of "verbal and symbolic acts" expected to cause psychological harm, with raw scores ranging from 0 to 117. The physical assault scale represents the amount of physical abuse in an intimate relationship, with raw scores ranging from 0 to 61. Finally, the injury scale indicates the amount of injuries that occurred as a result of IPV, with raw scores ranging from 0 to 4.

Each participant was asked to rate a series of statements about their mothers' and fathers' (or stepmothers' and stepfathers') relationship when they were approximately 12 years old. They were also given the option of endorsing any item that occurred prior to or after the age of 12. Any endorsement that happened before or after the stipulated age was tallied and recorded.

The Detailed Assessment of Posttraumatic Stress (DAPS)

The DAPS was used to assess the amount of trauma that participants perceived to result from exposure to IPV and to screen for Acute Stress Disorder (ASD) and Post-traumatic Stress Disorder (PTSD) (*Briere,*

TABLE 1. Demographic information about individual participants

Name*	Sex	Age	Ethnicity	Education Status	Employment Status	Annual Household Income	Relationship Status	Length of Relationship	Number of Children
Marissa	F	26	Caucasian	College Graduate	Part-Time/Student	Under $15,000	Living Together, Unmarried	5 years	0
Josie	F	27	Caucasian	Master's Degree	Part-Time	$31,000–$50,999	Living Together, Unmarried	1 year 6 months	1
John	M	28	Caucasian	College Graduate	Full-Time	$51,000–$99,999	Living Together, Unmarried	1 year 6 months	0
Claire	F	27	Caucasian	Master's Degree	Part-Time/ Student	$31,000–$50,999	Living Together, Unmarried	3 years 6 months	0
Peter	M	35	Latino	Some College	Student	Under $15,000	Dating, Not Living Together	5 years	2
Cindy	F	32	Caucasian	Master's Degree	Part-Time/ Student	$51,000–$99,999	Married	4 years	0
Kirsten	F	31	Caucasian	Master's Degree	Full-Time/ Student	Under $15,000	Dating, Not Living Together	1 year	0
Roseanne	F	31	Caucasian	College Graduate	Unemployed	$31,000–$50,999	Married	15 years	0
Lydia	F	35	African-American	Some College	Full-Time	$31,000–$50,000	Married	10 years	2
Gina	F	23	Caucasian	High School Graduate	Full-Time	$51,000–$99,999	Married	4 years	0

*All names have been changed to maintain confidentiality.

2001). The measure consists of 104 statements and takes approximately 20–30 minutes to complete. Respondents are asked to select one of five categories ranging from *"in the last day"* to *"a year ago or longer"* based on the time that is most accurate for each statement. The DAPS is composed of 2 validity and 11 clinical scales. It also includes three PTSD symptom clusters (re-experiencing, avoidance, hyperarousal) and three associated features of PTSD (dissociation, substance abuse, suicidality) related to a particular traumatic event. Results on the DAPS produce a provisional diagnosis of PTSD or ASD based on the *Diagnostic and Statistical Manual of Mental Disorders* (APA, 2000) criteria.

Personality Assessment Screener (PAS)

The PAS was used to assess for normative mental health, and was developed by Morey as both a brief assessment of mental health and a tool to identify clinical issues *Morey, 1997*. It consists of 22 items, each assessing the degree to which a particular symptom has caused discomfort in the respondent. Symptom distress is rated on a four-point Likert scale ranging from *"false"* to *"very true."* The items generate a total score and 10 "element" subscales that correspond to psychological symptoms including: negative affect, psychotic features, suicidal thinking, anger control, acting out, social withdrawal, alienation, health problems, hostile control, and alcohol problems. High scores indicate a high likelihood of problematic psychological functioning in the participant. Any score above 50 is considered in the clinical range (Morey, 1997). Raw scores on the PAS were converted into P-scores. A P-score of 50 or more indicates that a person has a 50% chance of exhibiting some type of clinical problems. For the purpose of the current study, a person who exhibited normative mental health was considered resilient.

The Michigan Alcoholism Screening Test (MAST) and the Drug Abuse Screening Test (DAST)

The MAST and DAST were used to assess for alcohol abuse and abuse of prescription and illegal drugs, respectively, in the past 12 months; (Selzer, 1971; Skinner, 1982). The MAST consists of 25 items and the DAST 28 items measured on dichotomous (yes/no) scales. The MAST is scored by adding the points for each "yes" answer. Items are weighted and behaviors or feelings that are especially indicative of a problem with alcohol are weighted more heavily. An overall score of three or less indicates no difficulties with alcohol, while a score of four indicates possible alcoholism and a score of five or more is indicative of alcoholism (Selzer, 1971). For the DAST, the total score is achieved by adding all endorsed items in the direction of drug abuse problems within the past 12 months. Each item is weighted equally, and total scores can range from 0 to 28, with higher scores indicating a greater degree of problems with drug abuse. Individuals scoring five points or more are very likely to be substance abusers or substance dependent. For the purpose of the current study, a person who did not have an alcohol or substance abuse problem was considered resilient.

Procedures

Flyers were placed around college campuses in San Diego, California, as well as free and paid advertisements in local newspapers. Potential participants voluntarily completed a demographic screener/questionnaire. Individuals who qualified were then invited to participate. A total of 121 people were screened and 19 qualified for further participation in the study. Of the 19 qualifying participants, three missed their scheduled appointments (one declined to reschedule and two could not be contacted to reschedule) and six did not meet the established criteria based on the written measures, resulting in 10 participants who met eligibility criteria.

After completion of the eligibility screening measures, eligible participants completed a semi-structured, in-depth interview. Interview topics included the participant's experiences of exposure to IPV as a child and the internal/individual characteristics, family, and external factors that contributed to his/her resilience. Interview questions were based on themes suggested by the literature regarding resilience. After completion of the interview, each participant was verbally debriefed. At the end of debriefing, interview participants received a $50 incentive. All procedures were reviewed and approved by the Institutional Review Board at the California School of Professional Psychology at Alliant International University.

RESULTS

Eligibility Screening

Table 2 depicts the scores of each participant on the CTS2-CA. Based on a clinical interpretation of these data, results indicate that all participants were exposed to IPV as children. Table 3 displays participants'

TABLE 2. Description of individual participant raw scores revised conflict tactics scale (Form CA)

	Marissa	Josie	John	Claire	Peter	Cindy	Kirsten	Roseanne	Lydia	Gina
Mother Negotiation	60	120	86	21 1*	33	88	42	17 3*	68	68
Father Negotiation	60	120	47	19 1*	8 1*	88	7	32 3*	8	49
Mother Psychological Aggression	117	0 6*	63	78	59	51 3*	1	40 1*	57	89
Father Psychological Aggression	65	0 5*	87	76	26	44 3*	41	30 2*	81	103
Mother Physical Assault	10	0 5*	1	12	30	0 8*	0	0	12 1*	61 3*
Father Physical Assault	9 2*	0	33	15	12 3*	0 10*	5	4 3*	21	51 1*
Mother Injury	2 2*	0	0	6 1*	3	0 5*	1 1*	0 2*	7	8 1*
Father Injury	2 1*	0 1*	0	4 1*	0	0 5*	0	0 1*	1	2 1*

*Indicates number of items endorsed for lifetime, but not in that year.

TABLE 3. The detailed assessment of post-traumatic stress description of individual scores on validity and clinical scales

	Marissa	Josie	John	Claire	Peter**	Cindy	Kirsten	Roseanne	Lydia**	Gina
Validity Scales										
PB	36	52	28	41	38	31	31	62	100+**	41
NB	46	46	55	46	88**	46	46	46	46	46
Clinical Scales										
RTE	40	40	51	45	60	58	40	45	40	58
PDST	63	75*	75*	37	70*	75*	65*	41	71*	73*
PDIS	42	73*	68*	42	53	53	61	42	65*	57
RE	52	56	78*	46	46	48	46	46	87*	56
AV	48	51	63	48	46	50	44	44	70*	48
AR	51	51	68*	44	45	49	44	47	46	48
PTS-T	50	53	70*	46	46	49	44	46	85*	50
IMP	48	62	59	57	53	45	45	45	66*	45
T-DIS	54	47	58	47	47	47	47	47	77*	47
SUB	69*	52	70*	47	70*	58	47	58	47	64
SUI	47	47	51	47	47	47	47	47	47	50

*Clinically significant. Clinical significance is a T-score of 65 or more.
**Protocols may be invalid due to inflated validity scale scores.

T-scores on the DAPS scales. Of the 10 participants, none met the criteria for a diagnosis of either PTSD or ASD.[1] Several of the participants did, however, experience some type of trauma as a result of the exposure to IPV. Seven of the participants' T-scores were clinically significant in the Peritraumatic Distress scale (PDST; T-scores 65–75), indicating that the individual experienced emotional and cognitive stress during the time of the traumatic event. Three participants endorsed items for the Peritraumatic Dissociation scale (PDIS), suggesting that the individuals dissociated during the traumatic event. P-scores on the PAS ranged from 5.7 to 48.9, with a mean of P-score of 31. The scores for Kirsten and Roseanne (P-scores of 5.7 and 14.1, respectively) indicated that it is unlikely that they have any identifiable clinical problems. Lastly, participants' scores on the MAST and DAST ranged from 0–3, indicating that substance or alcohol abuse issues were unlikely.

Major and Minor Research Findings Based on Interviews

The results of the qualitative analyses of the interview data yielded major and minor themes that were grouped into three categories. These categories included internal factors/individual characteristics, family factors, and external factors. Major themes were defined as being endorsed by 80% or more of the participants, and minor themes were endorsed by 50–70% of the participants.

Internal Factors/Individual Characteristics

Planning and Pursuing Goals

Nine participants viewed themselves as oriented to achieving future goals. They were optimistic and hopeful of the future and planned to achieve their personal and professional objectives. Josie and Roseanne indicated that planning for the future was their way of creating structure and having a stable environment. In fact, Roseanne believed her unstable childhood experiences may have carried over into her adult life and now she "wants everything to be very stable, very goal-oriented, organized."

Academic Success

Nine participants reported that they were successful academically. The demographic information obtained from the participants provided some supporting evidence for this factor. All 10 participants had finished high school, two completed some college, three were college graduates, and four earned Master's degrees. The participants also valued education as a way to improve their lives, and indicated that they were smart. Marissa, Cindy, and Roseanne stated that they were in accelerated classes, while Josie, Kirsten, and Gina reported that they experienced educational difficulties but had managed to overcome those challenges. These two opposing experiences exemplified the complexity of this factor. A person may feel adept because they earn high grades or they may feel proficient because they met and exceeded expectations despite the learning difficulties. In either case, the participants believed that their academic success was a factor to their resilience.

Internal Locus of Control

An internal locus of control was identified as important by eight participants. They described having control and structure in their lives. Additionally, the participants attributed their success to their perseverance and hard work. They also reported that they often felt unstable and encountered unpredictable family situations when growing up. Thus, it is reasonable to consider that they felt the need to control their environments in order to maintain stability in their lives.

Regulating Emotions

Eight participants reported that they adequately controlled their emotional states and were able to do so with relative ease. In particular, they believed that it was easier to control positive feelings rather than negative emotions. For example, Marissa, Gina, and Kirsten disclosed that it was difficult to manage their anger. The participants described avoiding negative emotional experiences, especially feelings they associated with the IPV (e.g., anger), and did not believe that they handled those feelings adequately. Thus, these individuals were focused on maintaining a more stable emotional state.

Generally Positive Perception of Self

Many participants described having generally positive self-perceptions. Additionally, they characterized their self-esteem as usually high or adequate. They demonstrated their confidence in a variety of professional and personal situations. For the participants, having a strong sense of self was related to overall positive perceptions of their persona. These individual characterized themselves as caring, sensitive to others, intelligent, easygoing, good-humored, and light-hearted. Additionally, these favorable characteristics were associated with other protective factors identified during their interviews. For example, Marissa identified being intelligent and reported that she experienced a high degree of academic success, which then reinforced her positive self-image.

Learning from Past Experiences

The aggression experienced in childhood was not a strong reinforcer for the adults in this study, and eight participants shared how they had learned from their past experiences. Although Claire, Cindy, and Kirsten admitted having abusive relationships in the past, their current intimate relationships were not violent. In fact, participants who endorsed this theme suggested that they did not desire to behave or observe their partner engaging in a manner similar to the IPV to which they were exposed during childhood. Each individual described how they made a strong commitment not to engage in IPV.

Family Factors

Closeness to Someone in their Family of Origin

Despite childhood exposure to IPV, nine participants stated that they were close to a member of their families of origin. Two of these nine individuals identified a general closeness in their families of origin. Seven participants were close to a parent, while five reported being connected to a sibling. Kirsten described being particularly close to her mother when her father acted out aggressively. Some participants identified characteristics of respect and nurturing in their relationships with family members. For example, Cindy appreciated the care and availability of her mother. Thus, it appears that closeness to a family member is an essential buffer for adults exposed to IPV as children.

Physical Distance from Family of Origin

Six participants revealed that physically distancing themselves from their families of origin was important to their positive adjustment. This minor theme presents potentially new information about resilience among adults exposed to IPV as children. It appears logical that these individuals needed to individuate from their families of origin. In fact, Peter and Kirsten specifically addressed separation and individuation. Another reason for removing themselves physically from their families of origin was a means to create and maintain manageable boundaries with their parents.

For example, Claire reinforced her decision to move 3000 miles away from her parents and added that she was in control of how much time she invested speaking with her parents.

This theme interacted with others presented previously, particularly the internal factors or individual characteristics. High self-esteem and positive perceptions of self are concepts associated with the task of developing a strong sense of self while separating and individuating from the family of origin. Having an internal locus of control is a factor that relates to being able to manage relationships with family members while maintaining a sense of self. Thus, individuation from family members appears to be an important feature to the resilient process.

Accepting Family of Origin Imperfections

The ability to accept flaws in their families of origin was a factor endorsed by six participants. These individuals recognized the imperfections of their parents and their parents' relationship. This finding is interesting as it demonstrates a unique concept associated with resilience among adults exposed to IPV as children. That is, participants demonstrated the ability to evaluate and accept the imperfections in their families of origin while developing a sense of self separate from them. For example, Marissa shared that while she did not always understand her parents' relationship, she felt a part of the family.

Retaining Family of Origin Values

Five participants reported that they maintained values that they learned from their families of origin. Evaluating the beliefs learned from the family of origin is a component of developing autonomous values. For example, Josie recognized that her orientation toward future goals was directly related to being raised in an environment that values pursuing goals. Thus, retaining family of origin values is connected to the development of a sense of self that is related to the process of resilience among adults exposed to IPV as children.

Developing a Closer Relationship with a Parent

Reconnecting with a parent was identified by five participants as a positive step in their development. For example, Gina described confronting her father about her negative experiences in childhood. Through this open dialogue, she was able to reconnect with her father and increase a level of emotional intimacy.

External Factors

Social Support System

Probably the most significant finding in the current study is that all 10 participants addressed the importance of a social support system. They felt secure in their relationships with others and described maintaining stable friendships. Social support is a critical component to resilience for several reasons. First, the individual searches for support outside the more unstable and volatile family system. For example, Cindy recognized that her friends were the support that she created outside her family of origin. Additionally, developing peer relationships provides an opportunity to experience different beliefs and values from those of the family of origin. Marissa identified having friends "who came from totally different places. . . . very different lives" and found it a fascinating aspect of her relationships. Peer relationships also allowed for the free expression of emotional experiences. For instance, Gina reported that her peer relationships gave her the chance to communicate her feelings freely. The ability to obtain alternative opinions and advice is another feature of social support networks. Lydia characterized her peer relationships as honest; she and her friends were able to share opposing viewpoints during their conversations. Lastly, peer relationships provided a secure and stable environment for individuals. For example, Claire reported that she trusts her friends "incessantly."

Important Adult Figures in Childhood

Another external factor that emerged was the presence of a positive adult figure in childhood. Nine participants described extended family members, teachers, coaches, and friends' parents as instrumental adults in their childhood. Some viewed the adult figures in their lives as role models for parenting and strength. Additionally, the adults present during their childhoods also modeled healthy relationship interactions.

Spiritual Beliefs

Nine participants reported having spiritual beliefs that allowed them to feel more connected to themselves and others. Spirituality was also considered a foundational component to their understanding of themselves and their interactions with their environment. A spiritual belief system is an important factor to resilience because it strengthens the perception of self. For example, Peter disclosed that he meditates in order to be more aware of himself and to hear his "inner voice." Spiritual beliefs are also important structures for individuals who experience adversity. Josie stated that her religion, Judaism, provided a structure for self-growth. Additionally, spiritual beliefs are used to connect with others. For instance, Cindy reported that her spirituality allowed her to connect with other people and help them on their lifelong paths.

Extracurricular Activities

This factor was noted by seven participants as instrumental to their resilience. The extracurricular activities described by participants included after-school activities, sports, and art. These activities increased self-esteem, were positive reinforcements, and were ways to escape from their families of origin. Internal factors or individual characteristics such as a positive perception of self or internal locus of control are seemingly related to outside interests. For example, Marissa described that her involvement in artistic expression assisted her in developing competencies and increased her self-esteem. It is reasonable to assume that extracurricular activities also link with other protective factors previously mentioned that promote resilience among adults exposed to IPV as children.

DISCUSSION

The present study increased our understanding of resilience among individuals exposed to IPV as children. A significant finding was the ability of the participants to learn from previous experiences and to change their behaviors and attitudes as they grew up. This concept is a central feature of resilience. It represents the ability to find meaning and live productively in spite of experiencing adversity (Werner, 1990). One of the main reasons the participants seemed to be resilient to the trauma was their ability to regulate emotions during their development. This major theme may also relate to having an internal locus of control for these individuals. Future research in this area of resilience may be able to delineate the relationship between regulating emotions and having an internal locus of control among adults exposed to IPV as children.

In addition, all 10 participants identified having a social support network as an important feature to their resilience. This protective factor is an established component of resilience and has been identified in multiple studies for other areas of childhood trauma (Parappully, Rosenbaum, Van

Den Daele, & Nzewi, 2002; Valentine & Feinauer, 1993; Werner, 1990). However, specific ways to promote the use of this factor have yet to be explored for children exposed to IPV. It would be helpful to determine ways to promote social support for such children in schools or in clinical settings.

A prevention approach based on the present findings could be useful in developing programs to promote resilience among children currently exposed to IPV. Treatment with children can be implemented in individual, family, and group therapy modalities. As 60% of violent men reported being exposed to IPV as children (Delsol & Margolin, 2004), it is also important to intervene early to prevent the intergenerational transmission of abuse. Clinical treatment should include interventions with offenders, victims, and their children. New assessment tools that measure resilience among individuals who experience adversities are expected to assist with clinical intervention by identifying strengths at early ages (Tedeschi & Kilmer, 2005). These measures can be implemented in addition to recommended treatment in order to foster resilience among these individuals. Lastly, understanding the perceived trauma associated with exposure to IPV is also necessary in order to provide appropriate therapeutic interventions with this population.

The purpose of using the DAPS in the present study was to collect collateral information about participants' perceived level of trauma. The information provided from the DAPS indicates that exposure to IPV can be cognitively and emotionally distressing to individuals, as indicated by high T-scores on the PDST and PDIS scales. These findings suggest that individuals exposed to IPV have unique needs that should be addressed during treatment.

Limitations of the Research

Due to the small sample size and qualitative nature of this study, the present findings cannot be generalized to the larger population nor do they allow for group comparisons (e.g., men versus women). The use of qualitative methods also precludes interpreting causality based on the results. Participants were mainly Caucasian and all were heterosexual; future research should thus explore resiliency and protective factors among racial, ethnic, and sexual minority groups. This study was based on a voluntary, self-selected population and therefore not representative of the demographics of the general population of California or the United

States. Finally, this study depended upon the participants' recollection of events from their childhood; such retrospective recall could result in memory biases or inaccuracies.

Strengths of the Research

Despite the limitations, this study enhanced the current literature pertaining to resilience. More specifically, this research explored the protective factors associated with resilience among adults exposed to IPV as children. To date, there are few, if any, studies that specifically investigated protective factors associated with resilience in this population. Most research in this area has examined resilience with individuals exposed to a variety of other adversities and traumas, such as maltreated or at-risk children (Werner & Smith, 2001).

To date, the information about the long-term effects of exposure to IPV in later adulthood has focused on negative trajectories, such as the intergenerational cycle of violence (Delsol & Margolin, 2004). Margolin (2005) suggested that future research investigate individuals who experience alternative developmental pathways. The present study investigated individuals who had positive outcomes despite being exposed to IPV and examined the protective factors they identified that contributed to their resilience. The findings of this qualitative research provide areas of focus for future research.

SUGGESTIONS FOR FUTURE RESEARCH

The present findings provide a foundational component to understanding this phenomenon, and future research may provide a more comprehensive awareness of resilience in this population. Future qualitative research should explore the key resilience and protective factors present in more racially, ethnically, and sexually diverse populations. In addition, the major and minor themes that emerged in this study should be tested quantitatively with a larger sample to examine whether the protective factors identified will hold up in other adults exposed to IPV as children. Finally, once the validity of these themes has been more established, it will be important to develop and implement therapeutic techniques that utilize and enhance these factors among individuals from a variety of different adverse experiences in childhood.

NOTE

1. It should be noted that two of the protocols in the current study may be invalid due to inflated scores on the DAPS' validity scales. Peter had an elevated score on the negative bias scale, suggesting that he presented himself in an overly symptomatic way (T-score = 88). Lydia had an elevated T-score on the positive bias scale, suggesting that she responded in a defensive manner (T-score = 100+). While the normative sample of the DAPS was comparable in ethnicity and race to the larger population (Briere, 2001), it is important to note that the two invalid profiles in this study were from Latino and African-American participants. It is uncertain if this measure is culturally sensitive and to date there is no information about the validity of the DAPS with ethnic or racial groups. However, data from these two participants were included in the study despite the elevated validity scores because the results from the PAS indicated that they were most likely not experiencing any clinical problems.

REFERENCES

American Psychiatric Association (APA). (2000). *Diagnostic and statistical manual of mental disorders* (4th ed.). Washington, DC: Author.

Briere, J. (2001). *Detailed assessment of posttraumatic stress (DAPS)*. Odessa, FL: Psychological Assessment Resources.

Carlson, B. E. (1984). Children's observations of interparental violence. In A. R. Roberts (Ed.), *Battered women and their families* (pp. 147–167). New York: Springer.

Delsol, C., & Margolin, G. (2004). The role of family-of-origin violence in men's marital violence perpetration. *Clinical Psychology Review, 24*, 99–122.

Fantuzzo, J. W., & Mohr, W. K. (1999). Prevalence and effects of children exposure to domestic violence. *The Future of Children: Domestic Violence and Children, 9*, 21–32.

Gewirtz, A. H., & Medhanie, A. (2008). Proximity and risk in children's witnessing of intimate partner violence incidents. *Journal of Emotional Abuse, 8*(1/2), 67–82.

Heller, S. S., Larrieu, J. A., D'Imperio, R., & Boris, N. W. (1999). Research on resilience to child maltreatment: Empirical considerations. *Child Abuse & Neglect, 23*, 321–338.

Kantor, G. K., & Jasinski, J. L. (1998). Dynamics and risk factors in partner violence. In J. L. Jasinski & L. M. Williams (Eds.), *Partner violence: A comprehensive review of 20 years of research* (pp. 73–112) Thousand Oaks, CA: Sage Publications.

Kracke, K., & Hahn, H. (2008). The nature and extent of childhood exposure to violence: What we know, why we don't know more, and why it matters. *Journal of Emotional Abuse, 8*(1/2), 29–49.

Margolin, G. (2005). Children's exposure to violence: Exploring developmental pathways to diverse outcomes. *Journal of Interpersonal Violence, 20*, 72–81.

Masten, A. S. (2001). Ordinary magic: Resilience processes in development. *American Psychologist, 56*, 227–238.

Miller-Perrin, C. L., & Perrin, R. D. (1999). *Child maltreatment: An introduction*. Thousand Oaks, CA: Sage Publications.

Morey, L. C. (1997). *Personality assessment screener professional manual*. Odessa, FL: Psychological Assessment Resources.

Osofsky, J. D. (2003). Prevalence of children's exposure to domestic violence and child maltreatment: Implications for prevention and intervention. *Clinical Child and Family Psychology Review, 6*, 161–170.

Parappully, J., Rosenbaum, R., Van Den Daele, L., & Nzewi, E. (2002). Thriving after trauma: The experiences of parents of murdered children. *Journal of Humanistic Psychology, 42*, 33–70.

Rutter, M. (1993). Disadvantage, resilience, and mature defenses. In G. E. Vaillant (Ed.), *The wisdom of the ego* (pp. 284–325). Cambridge, MA: Harvard University Press.

Selzer, M. L. (1971). The Michigan alcoholism screening test: The quest for a new diagnostic instrument. *American Journal of Psychiatry, 127*, 1653–1658.

Skinner, H. A. (1982). The drug abuse screening test. *Addictive Behaviors, 7*, 363–371.

Straus, M. A. (1992). Children as witnesses to marital violence: A risk factor for lifelong problems among a nationally representative sample of American men and women. In D. F. Schwarz (Ed.), *Children and violence: Report of the Twenty-Third Ross Roundtable on Critical Approaches to Common Pediatric Problems in Collaboration with the Ambulatory Pediatric Association* (pp. 98–109). Columbus, OH: Ross Laboratories.

Straus, M. A., Hamby, S. L., & Warren, W. L. (2003). *The Conflict Tactics Scale handbook, revised CTS (CTS2) and CTS parent-child version (CTSPC)*. Los Angeles: Western Psychological Service.

Tedeschi, R.G., & Kilmer, R. P. (2005). Assessing strengths, resilience, and growth to guide clinical interventions. *Professional Psychology: Research and Practice, 36*, 230–237.

Valentine, L., & Feinauer, L. L. (1993). Resilience factors associated with female survivors of childhood sexual abuse. *The American Journal of Family Therapy, 21*, 216–224.

Walsh, F. (1998). *Strengthening family resilience*. New York: The Guilford Press.

Werner, E. E. (1990). Protective factors and individual resilience. In S. J. Meisels & J. P. Shonkoff (Eds.), *Handbook of early childhood intervention* (pp. 97–116). New York: Cambridge University Press.

Werner, E. E., & Smith, R. S. (2001). *Journeys from childhood to midlife: Risk, resilience, and recovery*. Ithaca, NY: Cornell University Press.

Examination of Sex Differences and Type of Violence Exposure in a Mediation Model of Family Violence

Nicolette L. Howells
Alan Rosenbaum

A great deal of attention has been paid to the effects of a violent family environment on children. In 1981, Rosenbaum and O'Leary (1981) first used the term "unintended victims" to capture the idea that children in homes in which intimate partner aggression was occurring were at risk not only for psychological, emotional, and behavioral difficulties as children, but also for subsequently perpetrating aggression in their own adult intimate relationships. Numerous studies have since demonstrated that children or adolescents experiencing violence show elevated levels of externalizing behaviors, such as aggression (Christopoulos et al., 1987; Holden & Ritchie, 1991; Kaufman & Cicchetti, 1989; Rossman & Rosenberg, 1997), conduct problems (Hershorn & Rosenbaum, 1985; Rosenbaum & O'Leary, 1981), and other behavior problems (Hughes & Barad, 1983; Jaffe, Wolfe, Wilson, & Zak, 1986; Kolbo, 1996; Shahinfar, Fox, & Leavitt, 2000; Wolfe, Jaffe, Wilson, & Zak, 1985).

Children's exposure to psychological or verbal aggression or intimate partner violence (IPV) has been associated with feelings of anxiety and depression and subsequent aggressive behavior (Litrownik, Newton, Hunter, English, & Everson, 2003), including physical aggression in their relationships with their peers, dating partners, or parents (McCloskey & Lichter, 2003). A child's experience of being victimized by psychological and physical aggression in the home has also been significantly correlated with the child's subsequent aggressive behavior, anxiety, and depression (Litrownik et al., 2003). These studies exemplify several important issues. First, the term "experiencing violence in the family of origin" is used inconsistently (see Kracke & Hahn (2008, this issue) for a comprehensive discussion of definitional issues). It often refers to a child witnessing IPV, whether or not that child is actually present when the violence occurs. The term also subsumes the possibility of the child being a victim of child physical abuse (CPA). Given the co-occurrence rates of IPV and CPA, which Jaffe, Lemon, and Poisson (2003) place at 30–60%, it would appear to be important to account for this variable in terms of sample selection and description as well as in data analyses. A review of the literature reveals substantial variability across studies regarding whether this variable is considered. In some cases, researchers only report forms of violence that are the focus of the study (Boney-McCoy & Finkelhor, 1995; Kaplan et al., 1998; Kazdin, Moser, Colbus, & Bell, 1985), and it is unclear whether other forms of exposure may have occurred or were even assessed. This makes it difficult to attribute child problems to one or the other.

Second, exposure to various forms of aggression may be associated with behavioral problems, such as aggression and oppositional behavior;

and emotional problems, such as anxiety and depression. The fact that multiple forms of abuse frequently co-occur suggests the possibility of a relationship between type of exposure (IPV or CPA) and the nature of the sequellae (behavioral or emotional). Research in which the forms of exposure are differentiated has found that compared to non-IPV exposed and nonabused children, children who have both witnessed IPV and experienced CPA have lower self-esteem (Hughes, 1988), poorer social competence (Jaffe et al., 1986; Wolfe, Zak, Wilson, & Jaffe, 1986), poorer academic performance (Wolfe et al., 1986), and have shown higher problem scores (Hughes, 1988) such as depressive symptomology (Martin, Sigda, & Kupersmidt, 1998).

When compared to children who have only witnessed IPV, abused and IPV-exposed children have shown higher scores on measures of depressive symptomology (Martin et al., 1998), general psychopathology (McCloskey, Figueredo, & Koss, 1995), and behavior problems (O'Keefe, 1994), and lower scores on measures of sense of well-being (Carlson, 1991) and positive perceptions of their parents (Sternberg et al., 1993). Similar results were found when comparing children who are only victims of CPA to children who are both a witness to IPV and a victim of CPA, as children who experienced both types of violence reported higher levels of depressive symptomatology than those who had only experienced CPA (Martin et al., 1998). Children who only witnessed IPV fell in the middle of these groups, but were not significantly different than either (Hughes, Parkinson, & Vargo, 1989).

Overall, existing research suggests that the combination of witnessing IPV and experiencing CPA has more detrimental effects on children than experiencing either of these types of violence alone. However, one study found that children who had witnessed IPV only scored significantly higher on a measure of depressive symptomatology than children who had both witnessed IPV and experienced CPA and children who did not experience either type of violence (Hughes, 1988). While an overview of the literature confirms that many types of violence occurring in the family of origin may be sufficient to cause negative long-term effects (Kitzmann, Gaylord, Holt, & Kenny, 2003), future research must clarify the type of exposure being examined as well as the specific consequences for children exposed to the various types.

Much of the extant research on the effects of witnessing IPV or experiencing CPA has focused on children aged 5–12; however, studies that have used young adults have found many of the same effects as studies employing child samples, suggesting that the effects of experiencing some type of violence may be long term. For example, using college students,

Blumenthal, Neemann, and Murphy (1998) found that witnessing IPV was significantly associated with depression, anxiety, anger, interpersonal problems, and trauma symptoms. However, it was unclear if the authors controlled for the possibility of CPA. Among adult females who witnessed IPV during childhood, Henning, Leitenberg, Coffey, Turner, and Bennett (1996) found that the combination of witnessing IPV and experiencing CPA resulted in significantly more psychological distress than the sole occurrence of either witnessing IPV or experiencing CPA.

Gender Differences in Responses to Violence Exposure

Several studies have addressed the possibility that males and females may respond differently to family violence exposure. Girls who have witnessed IPV have been found to display more worry and oversensitivity than boys who witnessed IPV (Hughes & Barad, 1983). Other studies have used both females and males in order to conduct within and between sex comparisons: Forsstrom-Cohen and Rosenbaum (1985) found that females who witnessed IPV (and who had not been victims of CPA) were significantly more aggressive and more depressed than females who did not witness IPV, and were also significantly more depressed than males who had witnessed IPV. While these findings suggest gender differences regarding the effects of exposure to IPV, in their review of literature on the outcomes of experiencing CPA for children, Fantuzzo and Mohr (1999) note that some studies have found that gender makes no difference and others have found that males were more severely and negatively affected then females.

Aggression and Depression

Research has shown a strong positive correlation between depressive symptoms and aggression. This relationship has been empirically supported by research with children from third through sixth grade (Weiss & Catron, 1994), mentally retarded individuals (Reiss & Rojahn, 1993), female adult prison inmates (Varese, Pelowski, Riedel, & Heiby, 1998), and male batterers (Pan, Neidig, & O'Leary, 1994; Vivian & Malone, 1997). Further, there is evidence that this relationship may be stronger for women than for men. Bjork, Dougherty, and Moeller (1997), for example, found that depression scores for females, but not males, correlated positively with aggressive responses. Jack (2003) proposed that among depressed women, anger is the central emotion that they try to mute or keep from sharing in their relationships. Women may internalize anger because it has not been socially acceptable for them to express it, thus precipitating feelings of helplessness and depression (Jack, 2003). The 20 women in Jack's study who reported engaging in generally aggressive acts also self-reported depressive symptomatology. Similarly, McCloskey and Lichter (2003) found that females were six times more likely to aggress if they were also depressed, a finding not replicated among males.

Since depression and exposure to violence in the family of origin have both been associated with aggressive behavior, it makes sense to examine the pathways of these relationships. McCloskey and Lichter (2003) found that depression partially mediated the relationship between witnessing IPV and adolescent peer aggression, with witnessing IPV maintaining a direct effect on aggression. One limitation of this study, however, was that the authors only included peer aggression in their model, a form of aggression that has been previously shown to affect males more than females.

In sum, growing up in homes in which violence is occurring places children at risk for a host of emotional and behavioral problems. Prominent among these are depression, anger, and aggression. Depression and aggression co-occur with sufficient frequency in both the theoretical and empirical literatures that there is ample justification for testing a mediator model. There is evidence that witnessing IPV or experiencing CPA affects males and females differentially and that females may be more prone to depression-mediated aggression. In addition, exposure to IPV frequently co-occurs with experiencing CPA. Although both are pernicious, their independent and synergistic consequences must be sorted out.

The purpose of this study was to further examine the mediator model of aggression proposed by McCloskey and Lichter (2003) and to examine the differential effects due to gender of the participant. For the purposes of this article, no violence exposure refers to participants who reported no history of IPV exposure or CPA. Three central hypotheses were explored:

a. Depressive symptoms will serve as a mediator between generalized aggression and experiencing family violence (either IPV exposure or CPA).
b. This mediation model will be moderated by gender, as the model will be more significant for females than for males.
c. Four exposure-to-violence groups will display different levels of depressive symptoms and aggression, such that (i) those who were both witness to IPV and who experienced CPA (combined violence group) will show higher levels of depressive symptomatology and

aggression than the witness IPV-only, victim of CPA-only, and no violence exposure groups; and (ii) the witness IPV-only and victim of CPA-only groups will have significantly higher levels of depressive symptomatology and aggression than the no-violence exposure group but will not differ from each other on these measures.

METHOD

Participants

Participants were 360 students (197 males and 163 females) enrolled in Introduction to Psychology at a large midwestern university. Students participated voluntarily and received participation points, which was one way of satisfying a course research requirement. The ethnic composition of the sample was 50% Caucasian, 30.3% African American, 8.6% Hispanic, 6.4% Asian American, 0.3% Native American, and 4.2% other. The average age of the participants was 19.10 years (SD = 1.49). In addition, 73.6% of participants reported that as children, their major caregivers were both biological parents, 19.2% their biological mother only, 2.5% their biological father only, 1.4% their grandparents, and 3.3% other.

Measures

Conflict Tactics Scale – Revised (CTS2)

Experiencing family violence was measured using the physical assault and injury scales from the CTS2 (Straus, Hamby, Boney-McCoy, & Sugarman, 1996). Participants were asked to indicate how often they witnessed acts of violence between their parental figures, first with their male parental figure as the perpetrator of violence and a second time with their female parental figure as the perpetrator. Participants were then asked the same 17 items with themselves as the targets of the aggression and first their male parental figure and then their female parental figure as perpetrator. For the purposes of the study, scores from the male and female parental figures were added together for witnessing IPV and being physically abused. Internal consistency alpha coefficients for American undergraduate students on the physical assault subscale was .86 and the alpha coefficient for the injury subscale was .95 (Straus et al., 1996). The alpha coefficient for the overall measure in the present study was .95.

Beck Depression Inventory (BDI)

The BDI (Beck, Ward, Mendelson, Mock, & Erbaugh, 1961) is a 21-item, self-report measure of the characteristic attitudes and symptoms of depression. Scores range from 0 to 63, with those below 10 indicating no or minimal depression, scores from 10–18 indicate mild-to-moderate depression, scores from 19–29 indicate moderate-to-severe depression, and scores ranging from 30–63 indicate severe depression (Beck, Steer, & Garbin, 1988). The BDI has demonstrated validity and reliability (Foa, Riggs, Dancu, & Rothbaum, 1993; Richter, Werner, Heerlien, Kraus, & Sauer, 1998). Internal consistency alpha coefficients for American undergraduate students range from .78 (Golin & Hartz, 1979) to .87 (Lightfoot & Oliver, 1985). The alpha coefficient for the present study was .88.

Aggression Questionnaire (AQ)

The AQ (Buss & Perry, 1992) is a 29-item measure of four aspects of aggression: physical aggression, verbal aggression, anger, and hostility. Respondents rate how characteristic each item is of them on a scale of 1 (*extremely uncharacteristic of me*) to 5 (*extremely characteristic of me*). Questions about aggression toward others do not specify relationship or gender, so this instrument can capture both peer and dating aggression. The total AQ score provides an overall measure of aggressiveness and has a reported alpha of .89 (Buss & Perry, 1992). The alpha coefficient for the present study was .93. The AQ also shows adequate test-retest reliability (Buss & Perry, 1992).

Procedure

Institutional Review Board (IRB) approval for the study procedures was obtained before data collection began. Participants completed the CTS2, BDI, and AQ in groups ranging from 4 to 25. Participants were also asked four demographic questions regarding their gender, age, ethnicity, and who acted as their parental figures. The informed consent form was included as the first page in the questionnaire packet and was separated from the questionnaires to insure anonymity. Completed questionnaires were returned to the experimenter present in the room.

Statistical Analyses

Scores on the CTS2 were summed and used to classify participants into violence exposure groups. In testing the mediation hypotheses (Hypotheses A and B), in order to retain the variability necessary for regression, analyses participants were classified into an "experienced family violence" group if they endorsed any level of exposure to violence (i.e., if they had a score ranging from 1 to 32 on the CTS2; this group included those reporting IPV exposure only, those reporting CPA only, and those reporting both) or a "no family violence" group if they reported no history of either IPV exposure or CPA. In testing Hypothesis C, participants were classified based on their CTS2 scores into one of four groups: witness to IPV only, experiencing CPA only, both witness to IPV and experiencing CPA, and no exposure to violence. As previous research has shown that between 70–90% of parents spank their children at least occasionally (Saadeh, Rizzo, & Roberts, 2002), it was important to insure that the participants classified as victims were actually victims of child abuse. To be classified in the CPA group, participants had to report more than one occurrence on the questions regarding pushing and shoving, slapping, and grabbing. This classification affected each of the four exposure groups. For example, in some instances reporting only one occurrence of pushing and shoving, slapping, or grabbing resulted in a classification into the witness-only group if they had seen IPV or the no-exposure-to-violence group if they had not. There was a total of 143 participants in the no-exposure group, 21 in the witnessed IPV group, 92 in the victim of CPA group, and 99 in the group that had both witnessed IPV and experienced CPA.

RESULTS

The hypothesis that depression would mediate the association between experiencing family violence and aggression was tested using procedures outlined by Baron and Kenney (1986). Of note, the exposure to family violence variable was highly skewed ($M = 20.43$, $SD = 31.45$, skew = 2.73) as the majority of participants in the study reported no exposure to violence, and few had extremely high exposure to violence, which would be expected. As the skew of this variable was not corrected, results involving this variable should be interpreted cautiously.

Pearson r correlation analyses yielded significant associations between experiencing violence and depression, $r(360) = .221$, $p < .001$; violence and aggression, $r(360) = .285$, $p < .001$; and depression and aggression, $r(360) = .410$, $p < .001$. Multiple step-wise regression analyses were then conducted to examine the relationship between experiencing violence, depression, and aggression. For the first zero-order regression analysis, experiencing violence was significantly predictive of aggression, $F(1,356) = 31.52$, $p < .001$. For the second zero-order analysis, experiencing violence was significantly predictive of depression, $F(1,357) = 19.73$, $p < .001$. For the first step of the hierarchical regression analysis, depression was significantly predictive of aggression, $F(1,356) = 72.04$, $p < .001$. When the regression analyses were run to examine the effect of experiencing violence on aggression when taking into account the variability accounted for by depression, significance was again found, $F(2,355) = 46.65$, $p < .001$, suggesting that depression partially mediates the relationship between experiencing family violence and aggression. Sobel (1986) t-test analysis showed that depression served as a mediator between experiencing violence and aggression, $t(358) = 4.34$, $p < .001$. Standardized and unstandardized coefficients for each step are included in Table 1.

In order to test the second hypothesis, gender was introduced in the analysis to test whether it interacted with experiencing family violence in the mediation model. The model showed that gender moderated the relationship, $F(3, 329) = 29.84$, $p < .001$. To explain this moderation, the regression analyses were run to examine the relationship between experiencing violence, depression, and aggression for females only, and then for males only. For the first zero-order regression analysis, overall experiencing violence was significantly predictive of aggression for females, $F(1, 161) = 14.28$, $p < .001$, and for males, $F(1,193) = 17.37$, $p < .001$.

For the second zero-order regression analysis, overall experiencing violence was significantly predictive of depression for females, $F(1,161) = 14.48$, $p < .001$, and for males, $F(1,194) = 7.20$, $p = .008$. For the first step in the hierarchical regression analyses, depression was significantly predictive of aggression for females, $F(1, 161) = 70.04$, $p < .001$, and for

TABLE 1. Summary of hierarchical regression analyses for variables predicting aggressive behavior ($N = 360$)

Variable	B	SE B	β
Step 1			
Violence onto aggression	.20	.04	.29
Violence onto depression	.05	.01	.23
Step 2			
Depression onto aggression	1.30	.15	.41
Violence onto aggression	.15	.03	.21

$R^2 = .08$ for Step 1; $\Delta R^2 = .13$ for Step 2 ($p < .05$).

males, $F(1,193) = 18.78$, $p < .001$. When the Sobel t-tests were run to examine the significance of experiencing family violence on aggression, when taking into account the variability accounted for by depression, the analyses showed that depression partially, but significantly, mediated the relationship between experiencing violence and aggression for females, $t(160) = 3.41$, $p < .001$, but did not do so for males, $t(197) = 0.69$, $p = .49$. Standardized and unstandardized coefficients for each step for males are included in Table 2 and those for females are included in Table 3.

The effects of co-occurrence of the various forms of violence in the family of origin were examined in a 4 (type of violence exposure) × 2 (depressive symptoms and aggression) MANOVA. There was a significant main effect for group, Wilks' Lambda = 0.914, $F(3, 351) = 5.40$, $p < .001$. Univariate ANOVAs were then examined for each criterion variable,

TABLE 2. Summary of hierarchical regression analyses for variables predicting aggressive behavior for males ($N = 197$)

Variable	B	SE B	β
Step 1			
Violence onto aggression	.19	.05	.29
Violence onto depression	.04	.02	.19
Step 2			
Depression onto aggression	.93	.21	.30
Violence onto aggression	.16	.04	.24

$R^2 = .08$ for Step 1; $\Delta R^2 = .07$ for Step 2 ($p > .05$).

TABLE 3. Summary of hierarchical regression analyses for variables predicting aggressive behavior for females ($N = 163$)

Variable	B	SE B	β
Step 1			
Violence onto aggression	.22	.06	.29
Violence onto depression	.07	.02	.29
Step 2			
Depression onto aggression	1.79	.21	.55
Violence onto aggression	.11	.05	.14

$R^2 = .08$ for Step 1; $\Delta R^2 = .24$ for Step 2 ($p < .05$).

TABLE 4. Descriptives for groups included in post-hoc comparisons

Depression			Aggression		
Variable	Mean	SD	Variable	Mean	SD
No exposure	27.45	.57	No exposure	63.68	1.79
Witness IPV	27.29	1.48	Witness IPV	66.33	4.66
CPA	30.78	.71	CPA	76.12	2.23
Combined group	30.33	.68	Combined group	74.97	2.15

$N = 360$.

revealing significant results for depression, $F(3, 351) = 6.34$, $p < .01$, $\eta^2 = .051$, and aggression, $F(3, 351) = 8.69$, $p < .01$, $\eta^2 = .069$. A planned comparison Bonferroni analysis showed significant differences between the CPA victim-only and no-exposure groups ($p < .01$) and between the combined violence and the no-exposure and IPV witness-only groups ($p < .01$) for both depression and aggression. Table 4 includes means and standard deviations for each group included in the comparisons. Gender differences were not examined for this hypothesis due to the small number of participants in the IPV witness-only group.

DISCUSSION

Depressive symptoms served as a partial mediator between experiencing family (either IPV exposure or CPA) and aggression, with the experience of a form of family violence maintaining a direct effect on aggression (see also Samuelson & Cashman, 2008, this issue). This partially supported our hypothesis and was consonant with McCloskey and Lichter (2003), who found that depression partially mediated the relationship between exposure to family violence and adolescent peer aggression, with exposure to family violence maintaining a direct effect on aggression. This suggests that depression may serve as a partial mediator for both generalized as well as peer aggression.

The results also supported our hypothesis that the mediation model would be significant for females but not for males. One theory for the observed gender differences is the strong relationship between depressive symptoms and aggression for females (Bjork et al., 1997; Varese et al., 1998). However, it is also possible that depressive symptoms serve as a mediator between experiencing family violence and indirect aggression, which is seen more in females than males. Indirect, or relational, aggression is a form of aggression that involves attempts to harm others through the manipulation and ending of relationships and feelings of social inclusion (Crick & Grotpeter, 1995). Females may have been more likely to endorse indirect forms of aggression on the AQ, resulting in higher aggression scores. As the AQ does not specifically categorize items as indirect or direct aggression, future research should examine gender differences using a measure of indirect aggression as well as a measure of direct aggression.

The results provided only partial support for the third hypothesis. Contrary to expectations, the combined violence group did not report higher levels of depressive symptomatology and aggression than the CPA victim-only group, and the witness IPV-only group was not significantly different from the no-exposure group. These results suggest that experiencing CPA may be more important than witnessing IPV in producing the negative outcomes of exposure to family violence. There are a number of possible explanations for this finding. First, it may be the case that the intergenerational transmission of violence is more likely to occur when a child experiences CPA as opposed to watching someone else be victimized. Being a victim of CPA may thus be a stronger predictor of acting aggressively toward someone rather than only witnessing IPV. If modeling was the key to producing aggressive behavior, then it would be expected that witnessing IPV would also produce higher levels of aggression than a no-exposure group. However, this was not the case. Only participants who had both been victims of CPA and witnesses of IPV and those who had only been victims of CPA reported significantly higher levels of aggression than the no-exposure group. It may also be the case that exposure to different types of violence may predict different forms of aggression. For example, the dating violence research has shown that witnessing IPV predicts higher levels of aggression (Forsstrom-Cohen & Rosenbaum, 1985; Litrownik et al., 2003; McCloskey & Lichter, 2003). It may thus be possible that experiencing CPA is a stronger predictor of more generalized aggression. Further research is needed to clarify these relationships.

In the present study, one-third (34%) of participants recalled witnessing IPV. These numbers are comparable to the lifetime prevalence rate of violence in marriages (Gelles & Straus, 1988). The results in the present study also indicate that rates of co-occurrence of IPV exposure and CPA (28%) are comparable to those of CPA only (26%), and both exceed rates of IPV exposure alone (6%). These results suggest that if a child witnesses IPV in their home, there is a greater likelihood that they may also be experiencing CPA. However, experiencing CPA does not necessarily increase the likelihood of witnessing IPV. These results are consistent with research conducted by Margolin (1998), which found that more children are likely to report being victims of CPA if they are exposed to IPV than the opposite.

Limitations

This study had several limitations. First, depressive symptoms were measured for the 2 weeks prior to completion of the questionnaire. Although this is standard use of the BDI, depression was not measured prior to the occurrence of aggressive behavior. In addition, data for this study consisted of retrospective self-reports, introducing the possibility of a mono-method bias as well as recall bias. Future research would benefit from the addition of other data sources, such as interview or parent reports. Another limitation was the use of a convenience sample of college students, the majority of whom reported living with both biological parents.

The present study did not look into the chronicity of violence exposure or the age at which exposure occurred. In this study, participants were asked to report on any instances of exposure before age 18. Therefore, some participants may have been reporting on an event that occurred when they were 3 years old and others may have been reporting on incidents that occurred when they were 16 years old. Future research should look at the differences in outcomes based on the age at which exposure occurred, as well as the chronicity of the violence.

Clearly, exposure to violence in the family of origin is a complex constellation of variables. The present study moves beyond affirming the relationship between childhood exposure to violence and aggression to examining possible mechanisms by which exposure may produce aggression. Further, it confirms that the mechanisms may not be the same for both males and females. Information such as this is essential to both our understanding of aggression and our efforts to treat, and ultimately prevent, its occurrence.

REFERENCES

Baron, R. M., & Kenny, D. A. (1986). The moderator-mediator variable distinction in social psychological research: Conceptual, strategic, and statistical considerations. *Journal of Personality and Social Psychology, 51,* 1173–1182.

Beck, A. T., Steer, R. A., & Garbin, M. G. (1988). Psychometric properties of the Beck Depression Inventory: 25 years of evaluation. *Clinical Psychology Review, 8,* 77–100.

Beck, A. T., Ward, C. H., Mendelson, M., Mock, J., & Erbaugh, J. (1961). An inventory for measuring depression. *Archives of General Psychiatry, 4*, 561–571.

Bjork, J. M., Dougherty, D. M., & Moeller, F. G. (1997). A positive correlation between self-ratings of depression and laboratory-measured aggression. *Psychiatry Research, 69*, 33–38.

Blumenthal, D. R., Neemann, J., & Murphy, C. M. (1998). Lifetime exposure to interparental physical and verbal aggression and symptom expression in college students. *Violence and Victims, 13*, 175–196.

Boney-McCoy, S., & Finkelhor, D. (1995). Psychosocial sequelae of violent victimization in a national youth sample. *Journal of Consulting and Clinical Psychology, 63*, 726–736.

Buss, A. H., & Perry, M. (1992). The aggression questionnaire. *Journal of Personality and Social Psychology, 63*, 452–459.

Carlson, B. E. (1991). Outcomes of physical abuse and observation of marital violence among adolescents in placement. *Journal of Interpersonal Violence, 6*, 526–534.

Christopoulos, C., Cohn, D. A., Shaw, D. S., Joyce, S., Sullivan-Hanson, J. Kraft, S. P., et al. (1987). Children of abused women: I. Adjustment at time of shelter residence. *Journal of Marriage and the Family, 49*, 611–619.

Crick, N. R., & Grotpeter, J. K. (1995). Relational aggression, gender, and social-psychological adjustment. *Clinical Development, 66*, 710–722.

Fantuzzo, J. W., & Mohr, W. K. (1999). Prevalence and effects of child exposure to domestic violence. *The Future of Children: Domestic Violence and Children, 9*, 21–32.

Foa, E. B., Riggs, D. S., Dancu, C. V. S., & Rothbaum, B. O. (1993). Reliability and validity of a brief instrument for assessing post traumatic stress disorder. *Journal of Traumatic Stress, 6*, 459–473.

Forsstrom-Cohen, B., & Rosenbaum, A. (1985). The effects of parental marital violence on young adults: An exploratory investigation. *Journal of Marriage and the Family*, 467–472.

Gelles, R. J., & Straus, M. A. (1988). *Intimate violence*. New York: Simon & Schuster.

Golin, S., & Hartz, M. A. (1979). A factor analysis of the Beck Depression Inventory in a mildly depressed population. *Journal of Clinical Psychology, 35*, 323–325.

Henning, K., Leitenberg, H., Coffey, P., Turner, T., & Bennett, R. T. (1996). Long-term psychological and social impact of witnessing physical conflict between parents. *Journal of Interpersonal Violence, 11*, 35–51.

Hershorn, M., & Rosenbaum, A. (1985). Children of marital violence: A closer look at the unintended victims. *American Journal of Orthopsychiatry, 55*, 260–266.

Holden, G. W., & Ritchie, K. L. (1991). Linking extreme marital discord, child rearing, and child behavior problems: Evidence from battered women. *Child Development, 62*, 311–327.

Hughes, H. M. (1988). Psychological and behavioral correlates of family violence in child witnesses and victims. *American Journal of Orthopsychiatry, 8*, 77–90.

Hughes, H. M., & Barad, S. J. (1983). Psychological functioning of children in a battered women's shelter: A preliminary investigation. *American Journal of Orthopsychiatry, 53*, 525–531.

Hughes, H. M., Parkinson, D., & Vargo, M. (1989). Witnessing spouse abuse and experiencing physical abuse: A "double whammy"? *Journal of Family Violence, 4,* 197–209.

Jack, D. C. (2003). The anger of hope and the anger of despair. In J. M. Stoppard & L. M. McMullen (Eds.), *Situating sadness: Women and depression in social context* (pp. 62–87). New York: New York University Press.

Jaffe, P., Lemon, N., & Poisson, S. E. (2003). *Child custody and domestic violence: A call for safety and accountability.* Thousand Oaks, CA: Sage Publications.

Jaffe, P., Wolfe, D., Wilson, S. K., & Zak, L. (1986). Family violence and child adjustment: A comparative analysis of girls' and boys' behavior symptoms. *American Journal of Psychiatry, 143,* 74–77.

Kaplan, S. J., Pelcovitz, D., Salzinger, S., Weiner, M., Mandel, F. S., Lesser, M. L., et al. (1998). Adolescent physical abuse: Risk for adolescent psychiatric disorders. *American Journal of Psychiatry, 155,* 954–959.

Kaufman, J., & Cicchetti, D. (1989). Effects of maltreatment on school-age children's socioemotional development: Assessments in a day-camp setting. *Developmental Psychology, 25,* 516–524.

Kazdin, A. E., Moser, J., Colbus, D., & Bell, R. (1985). Depressive symptoms among physically abused and psychiatrically disturbed children. *Journal of Abnormal Psychology, 94,* 298–307.

Kitzmann, K. M., Gaylord, N. K., Holt, A. R., & Kenny, E. D. (2003). Child witnesses to domestic violence: A meta-analytic review. *Journal of Consulting and Clinical Psychology, 71,* 339–352.

Kolbo, J. R. (1996). Risk and resilience among children exposed to family violence. *Violence & Victims, 11,* 113–128.

Kracke, K., & Hahn, H. (2008). The nature and extent of childhood exposure to violence: What we know, why we don't know more, and why it matters. *Journal of Emotional Abuse, 8*(1/2), 29–49.

Lightfoot, S. L., & Oliver, J. M. (1985). The Beck Inventory: Psychometric properties in university students. *Journal of Personality Assessment, 49,* 434–436.

Litrownik, A. J., Newton, R., Hunter, W. M., English, D., & Everson, M. D. (2003). Exposure to family violence in young at-risk children: A longitudinal look at the effects of victimization and witnessed physical and psychological aggression. *Journal of Family Violence, 18,* 59–73.

Margolin, G. (1998). Effects of domestic violence on children. In P. K. Trickett & C. J. Shellenbach (Eds.), *Violence against children in the family and the community* (pp. 57–101). Washington, DC: American Psychological Association.

Martin, S. L., Sigda, K. B., & Kupersmidt, J. B. (1998). Family and neighborhood violence: Predictors of depressive symptomology among incarcerated youth. *Prison Journal, 78,* 423.

McCloskey, L. A., Figueredo, A. J., & Koss, M. P. (1995). The effects of systematic family violence on children's mental health. *Child Development, 66,* 1239–1261.

McCloskey, L. A., & Lichter, E. L. (2003). The contribution of marital violence to adolescent aggression across different relationships. *Journal of Interpersonal Violence, 18,* 390–412.

O'Keefe, M. (1994). Linking marital violence, mother-child/father-child aggression, and child behavior problems. *Journal of Family Violence, 9*, 63–78.

Pan, H. S., Neidig, P. H., & O'Leary, K. D. (1994). Predicting mild and severe husband-to-wife physical aggression. *Journal of Consulting and Clinical Psychology, 62*, 975–981.

Reiss, S., & Rojahn, J. (1993). Joint occurrence of depression and aggression in children and adults with mental retardation. *Journal of Intellectual Disability Research, 37*, 287–294.

Richter, P., Werner, J., Heerlien, A. Kraus, A., & Sauer, H. (1998). On the validity of the Beck Depression Inventory: A review. *Psychopathology, 31*, 160–168.

Rosenbaum, A., & O'Leary, K. D. (1981). Children: The unintended victims of marital violence. *American Journal of Orthopsychiatry, 51*, 692–699.

Rossman, B. B. R., & Rosenberg, M. S. (1997). Psychological maltreatment: A needs analysis and application for children in violent families. *Journal of Aggression, Maltreatment & Trauma, 1*, 245–262.

Saadeh, W., Rizzo, C. D., & Roberts, D. G. (2002). Spanking. *Clinical Pediatrics, 41*, 87–88.

Samuelson, K. W., & Cashman, C. (2008). Effects of intimate partner violence and maternal posttraumatic stress symptoms on children's emotional and behavioral functioning. *Journal of Emotional Abuse, 8*(1/2), 139–153.

Shahinfar, A., Fox, N. A., & Leavitt, L. A. (2000). Preschool children's exposure to violence: Relation of behavior problems to parent and child reports. *Journal of Orthopsychiatry, 70*, 115–125.

Sobel, M. E. (1986). Some new results on indirect effects and their standard errors in covariance models. In N. Tuma (Ed.), *Sociological methodology* (pp. 159–186). Washington, DC: American Sociological Association.

Sternberg, K. L., Lamb, M. E., Greenbaum, C., Cicchetti, D., Dawud, S., Cortes, R. M., et al. (1993). Effects of domestic violence on children's behavior problems and depression. *Developmental Psychology, 29*, 44–52.

Straus, M. A., Hamby, S. L., Boney-McCoy, S., & Sugarman, D. B. (1996). The Revised Conflict Tactics Scale (CTS2): Development and preliminary psychometric data. *Journal of Family Issues, 17*, 283–316.

Varese, T., Pelowski, S., Riedel, H., & Heiby, E. M. (1998). Assessment of cognitive-behavioral skills and depression among female prison inmate. *European Journal of Psychological Assessment, 14*, 141–145.

Vivian, D., & Malone, J. (1997). Relationship factors and depressive symptomology associated with mild and severe husband-to-wife physical aggression. *Violence and Victims, 12*, 3–18.

Weiss, B., & Catron, T. (1994). Specificity of the comorbidity of aggression and depression in children. *Journal of Abnormal Child Psychology, 22*, 389–401.

Wolfe, D. A., Jaffe, P., Wilson, S., & Zak, L. (1985). Children of battered women: The relation of child behavior to family violence and maternal stress. *Journal of Consulting and Clinical Psychology, 53*, 657–665.

Wolfe, D. A., Zak, L., Wilson, S., & Jaffe, P. (1986). Child witnesses to violence between parents: Critical issues in behavioral and social adjustment. *Journal Abnormal Child Psychology, 14*, 95–104.

Effects of Intimate Partner Violence and Maternal Posttraumatic Stress Symptoms on Children's Emotional and Behavioral Functioning

Kristin W. Samuelson
Caroline Cashman

One third of American children are estimated to have witnessed intimate partner violence (IPV) in their homes (Straus, 1992). IPV not only poses a threat to the physical health and psychological well-being of women involved in these violent relationships, but also threatens the well-being of children living in violent families. Reviews of research efforts documenting the impact of IPV on children have concluded that exposure to

IPV has a detrimental effect on children's functioning (Edelson, 1999; Fantuzzo & Lindquist, 1989; Fantuzzo & Mohr, 1999; Margolin & Gordis, 2000; also see Kracke & Hahn, this issue). Children exposed to IPV exhibit depression, aggressiveness and oppositionality, and problems with social, school, and cognitive functioning. Reviewers have cautioned that methodological problems, such as heterogeneity of the population, overreliance on samples of convenience (shelter samples), and poor discrimination of the constructs of child abuse and exposure to IPV, restrict the applicability of these findings (Edelson; Fantuzzo & Lindquist).

There are several possible explanations as to why children of battered women exhibit psychological problems. The first is that witnessing family violence is traumatic. Children who witness life-threatening violence between their parents are more likely to exhibit posttraumatic stress symptoms (PTSS) of their own (Pynoos & Eth, 1985). Alternatively, children of battered women may experience psychological problems because they are more likely to be maltreated themselves. In a review of IPV studies, Margolin (1998) found that between 45–70% of children exposed to IPV are also victims of physical abuse.

The third explanation is that IPV causes deleterious psychological consequences in the mother, making her less capable of caring for her children and responding to their needs. A history of IPV is associated with various psychological disorders that may interfere with a mother's relationship with her child, including depression, anxiety, personality disorders, substance abuse, and posttraumatic stress disorder (PTSD; Resnick & Acierno, 1997). Mothers, who are counted upon to provide nurturance and protection to their children, may be less able to do so when they are victims of violence, and it has been suggested that women with trauma histories may display impaired parenting skills (Hughes, 1982). These mothers are also likely to have difficulties attending to the emotional needs of their children. In their study of behavioral problems in children of battered women, Wolfe, Jaffe, Wilson, and Zak (1985) found that maternal stress variables accounted for 19% of the variance in children's behavioral functioning. Similarly, in a study of preschoolers living in neighborhoods with high rates of community violence, maternal distress mediated the relationship between child exposure to violence and child behavior problems (Linares et al., 2001). These studies support the notion that IPV can have an indirect impact on children's functioning through its effect on maternal functioning.

One of the most troubling mental health outcomes for battered women is PTSD. Studies have shown that 45–84% of battered women in community samples meet diagnostic criteria for PTSD (Astin, Lawrence, & Foy, 1993; Astin, Ogland-Hand, Coleman, & Foy, 1995). Symptoms of PTSD frequently found in battered women include re-experiencing symptoms such as intrusive thoughts, nightmares, and flashbacks; avoidance symptoms such as emotional numbing, feelings of detachment from others, and anhedonia; and hyperarousal symptoms such as sleep disturbance, hypervigilance, difficulty concentrating, and startle response (Saunders, 1994).

Relatively few studies have examined the impact of maternal PTSD on parenting and children's functioning. One exception, a study of battered women and their preschool-aged children (Lieberman, Van Horn, & Ozer, 2005), found that maternal PTSD mediated the relationship between maternal life stressors and child behavior problems. Chemtob and Carlson (2004) found that among mothers who had experienced IPV, those who had PTSD were more likely to be quick and impulsive in their actions toward their children. While some studies have examined the impact of trauma and PTSD on parenting and children's behavioral symptoms, no studies have examined the impact of maternal PTSD on emotion regulation difficulties in children. A child's ability to emotionally regulate is learned through interaction and dependent on the mother's ability to bond, connect, and provide a functional emotional regulatory model. The mother-child bond is thought to be a mechanism through which a child learns to self-soothe and modulate his/her own emotions (Cassidy, 1994), and if this bond is hindered by the mother's psychological health, then a child may be prevented from learning emotional regulation skills.

More evidence for the impact of parental PTSD on children is provided through studies of Vietnam veterans. While much of this research is focused on males with war-related PTSD, this substantial body of research provides valuable insight into the mechanisms by which parental PTSD affects children. In one study, children of veteran fathers with PTSD frequently exhibited symptoms similar to their fathers, such as symptoms of depression, anxiety, low frustration tolerance, and outbursts of anger (Harkness, 1993). Jordan and colleagues have documented elevated levels of family adjustment problems and poorer parenting skills in male Vietnam veterans (Jordan et al., 1992). Ruscio, Weathers, and King

(2002) examined the relationship between Vietnam veterans' PTSD symptomatology and their perceived quality of relationship with their children, finding that the avoidance cluster of PTSD most strongly related to perceived quality of relationship. These results suggest that emotional numbing and detachment, symptoms from the avoidance cluster, underlie parent-child relationship problems from the perspective of the parent. In their study of 250 male veterans designed to replicate and extend Ruscio et al.'s study, Samper, Taft, King, and King (2004) found that after controlling for depression, avoidance symptoms were associated with less parenting satisfaction and a poorer quality of parent-child relationship. These results suggest that emotional numbness associated with PTSD is distinct from emotional constriction sometimes found in depression.

These findings further build a case for the importance of studying emotion regulation in the children of parents with PTSD. Taken together, the results of these studies suggest that parents with PTSD may be emotionally disengaged and inaccessible to their children, less able to help their children form a secure attachment, and less able to teach them to modulate their affect and regulate their own emotions. This study seeks to further existing research by looking not only at exposure to IPV, but also maternal posttraumatic stress symptoms (PTSS) as predictors of child difficulties. Secondly, this study expands upon current research by exploring the hypothesis that maternal PTSS is associated with emotion regulation difficulties in the child, as well as child behavior problems.

METHODS

Participants

Participants were 30 women who had experienced IPV in the past but had not been in a violent relationship for at least six months, and who had at least one child between the ages of 5 and 18 years with whom they lived. Participants were recruited from the community, but not from shelters as added stressors in the shelter environment can impact both the mothers' and children's psychological adjustment. Participants were recruited through flyers posted at various community agencies throughout San Francisco and an advertisement on an online community message board. The sample was made up of 47% African-Americans, 37% Caucasians, 13% Hispanics, and 3% Asian Americans. The mean age of the participants was 39.5 years, with an age range from 23–58 years ($SD = 8.67$).

Participants had a mean of 2.3 children (SD = 1.4; range: 1–7 children). Mean education level was 14.57 years (SD = 2.03). Most participants were high school graduates (96.8%), most had some college education (90.3%), and 35% were college graduates. Fifty percent of the women were not employed, 13.3% were employed part time, and 36.7% were employed full time. Fifty percent of the women reported their annual income to be less than $20,000 a year, 27% between $20,000 and $40,000, and 23% over $40,000. The majority of the women (60%) were single, 27% were divorced, 10% were married, and 3% were widowed. All of the women reported that their batterers were men. Each mother was asked to answer questions about only one of her children. The women's children whom they reported on ranged in age from 5 to 18, with a mean age of 11.4 years (SD = 4.1). Eighteen of the children were male and 12 were female.

Procedure

Participants were interviewed about their experience of IPV and asked to complete a battery of self-report measures as well as parent-report measures about their children. Participation time ranged from 1–2.5 hours, and interviews were administered by clinical psychology graduate students. Participants were paid $25 for their participation and received referrals to various local agencies for follow-up support.

Because of the sensitive nature of the interview questions, informed consent included a statement that if it were revealed during the interview that the child had been harmed, the interviewer would contact appropriate authorities. Child Protective Services was consulted on three cases over the course of the study. Caseworkers informed the authors that two cases did not meet criteria for a filed report; a report was filed on the remaining case. Because parents were informed of the necessity to report child abuse, the actual prevalence of child maltreatment may be underrepresented in this sample.

Measures

Background Information Questionnaire

Participants were asked to provide personal data such as age, marital status, ethnicity, current occupation, level of education, household income, history of mental health interventions, number of children in the family, and the children's ages, as well as provide brief information about the violent relationship (their relationship to the batterer, his relationship to the children, and any legal consequences following the violence).

Conflict Tactics Scale 2 (CTS2)

The mother's experience of and the extent of IPV, as well as the child's degree of witnessing the IPV was assessed through the CTS2 (Straus, 1979; Straus, Hamby, Boney-McCoy, & Sugarman, 1996), a self-report questionnaire that assesses the occurrence and frequency of particular behaviors during interpersonal conflicts. The CTS2 has five subscales: Negotiation, Psychological Aggression, Physical Assault, Sexual Coercion, and Injury. Each question on the CTS2 asks the participant to indicate the frequency of the corresponding conflict resolution tactic on a seven-point Likert scale ranging from 0 (*never*) to 6 (*more than 20 times*). The CTS2 was administered as an interview, and the participants were asked to answer questions about their batterers' behaviors toward them and their children's experience of witnessing those behaviors (physical assault subscale only). The amount of IPV was obtained by scoring the midpoints of each response category in the physical assault subscale, according to the directions of the CTS2 manual (Straus et al.). The mothers also reported on both their own and the batterers' acts of abusive behaviors toward the target children. Internal reliability coefficients for the scale range from .79 to .95 (Straus et al.). In this study, reliability was high ($\alpha = .97$).

PTSD Checklist (PCL)

The mother's severity of PTSS was assessed through the PCL (Weathers, Litz, Herman, Huska, & Keane, 1993), a 17-item self-report measure that corresponds to the *Diagnostic and Statistical Manual of Mental Disorders* (DSM-IV; American Psychiatric Association, 1994) criteria for PTSD. The measure includes questions corresponding to the DSM-IV's five re-experiencing symptoms, seven avoidance and numbing symptoms, and five hyperarousal symptoms. Respondents are asked to indicate the extent to which they have been bothered by each symptom in the past month on a 5-point Likert scale ranging from 1 (*not at all*) to 5 (*extremely*). The PCL demonstrates excellent internal consistency (.94) and test-retest reliability (.88 for a one-week interval). Sensitivity in identifying PTSD ranges from 0.78 to 0.94 and specificity ranges from 0.83 to 0.86 (Blanchard, Jones-Alexander, Buckley, & Forneris, 1996). In this study, the internal reliability of this measure was .95.

Emotional Regulation Checklist (ERC)

Children's emotional functioning and regulation was assessed through the ERC (Shields & Cicchetti, 1997). The ERC is a 24-item measure of children's self regulation completed by the mother. Of interest to the present study was the Lability/Negativity subscale, which assesses processes including affective lability, angry reactivity, and emotional intensity. The internal reliability coefficient reported by the authors for this subscale was .96. Validity has been established through positive correlations with observers' ratings of children's self-regulatory abilities (Shields & Cicchetti). In this study, the internal reliability was .83 for the Lability/Negativity subscale.

Child Behavior Checklist (CBCL)

Children's behavioral functioning was assessed through the CBCL (Achenbach, 1991), a parental report measure of child psychopathology. The CBCL assesses for children's internalizing and externalizing symptoms on a 3-point scale ranging from 0 (*not true*) to 2 (*very true or often true*). This measure has high reliability and validity (Achenbach), and in this study, the internal reliability was .97.

Data Analysis

Bivariate correlations were conducted to examine the associations between demographic variables (mother and child's age, mother's education level, and income), child's witnessing of IPV, child's own maltreatment, mother's PTSS, and child's emotional and behavioral functioning. *T*-tests examined differences between child's ethnicity and gender on independent and dependent variables. Although multivariate analyses are cautioned against with a sample size this small, the presence of significant bivariate correlations suggests that hierarchical multiple regression analyses would be useful to assess the unique variance in child's mental health outcomes explained by mother's PTSS, above and beyond the extent of the child's own maltreatment of witnessing of IPV. Two hierarchical regression analyses were conducted, with ERC lability/negativity score and CBCL total score as the dependent variables, respectively. In each regression, any significant covariates were entered into the first step, the degree to which the child witnessed IPV was entered into the second step, the degree to which the child experienced maltreatment was entered into the third step, and mother's PTSS were entered into the final step.

RESULTS

Characteristics of the mothers and statistics regarding IPV histories are presented in Table 1. Of note, 53% of the mothers reported being physically or sexually abused as a child, and 57% had been in other violent intimate relationships. Ninety percent of the mothers had sought mental health services in their lifetime, and 10% had been hospitalized for psychiatric reasons. Sixty percent had sought mental health services for their children. Seventy-seven percent of the children witnessed IPV, while only 10% were maltreated themselves, according to mother's report. Forty-three percent of children witnessed severe physical violence, which included watching their mothers being punched, hit, choked, or burned.

There were no significant correlations between demographic variables (mother and child's age, mother's education level, income) and independent and dependent variables. There were no significant differences between children's ethnicities on any independent and dependent variables. There were gender differences on the CBCL total score, with girls ($M = 46.08$, $SD = 35.2$) scoring significantly higher than boys ($M = 26.0$, $SD = 17.5$), $t(28) = -2.03$, $p = .05$. Examining the subscales of the CBCL, this overall difference appears to be due to the significant difference between girls ($M = 12.00$, $SD = 9.45$) and boys ($M = 5.71$, $SD = 1.43$) on the Internalizing scale, $t(28) = -2.21$, $p = .036$, as there were no significant differences on the Externalizing scale.

TABLE 1. IPV and maltreatment histories of mothers and children

Characteristic	N	%
Mother abused as child	16	53
Other violent intimate relationships	17	57
Psychiatric services sought for self	37	90
Inpatient psychiatric hospitalization for mother	3	10
Psychiatric services sought for child	18	60
Verbal abuse experienced in relationship	30	100
Physical abuse experienced in relationship	28	93
Severe physical abuse experienced in relationship	25	83
Abuse involving injury experienced in relationship	23	77
Sexual abuse experienced in relationship	25	83
Physical abuse witnessed by child	23	77
Severe physical abuse witnessed by child	13	43
Child physically abused	3	10
Child Protective Services involvement	9	30

Correlational analyses revealed that childrens' emotional regulation difficulties were related to mothers' PTSS, $r = .68$, $p < .01$, and that children's internalizing and externalizing behaviors were also related to mothers' PTSS, $r = .60$, $p < .01$. Scores associated with amount of IPV witnessed were significantly related to CBCL scores, $r = .39$, $p < .05$, but not to emotional regulation difficulties. Correlations between child maltreatment and child outcome variables were also not significant; however, the potential underreporting of child maltreatment and the resultant small percentage of children in the sample (10%) with child maltreatment histories may affect this analysis.

Hierarchical multiple regression analyses were conducted to determine if mother's PTSS predicted child's mental health outcome, above and beyond the child's witnessing of violence and/or own maltreatment (see Table 2). Examining the Emotional Regulation/Negativity and Lability Index of the ERC as an outcome variable, extent of child witnessing was entered in the first step and was not a predictor of child's negative and labile emotion. The child's own maltreatment score, as measured by the CTS-2, was entered in the second step and was also not a significant predictor. Mother's PTSS severity was added in the third step and was a strong predictor of child's negative and labile emotion, R^2 *change* = .433, $\beta = .67$, $p < .001$, accounting for 43% of the variance in child's emotional regulation difficulties.

Examining total CBCL score as an outcome variable (see Table 3), child's gender was entered first into the regression model and explained a significant amount of the variance in child's behavior, $R^2 = .133$, $\beta = .364$,

TABLE 2. Hierarchical regression analysis for variables predicting children's emotional regulation/negativity and lability

Variable	B	SE B	β	p	95% CI
Step 1					
Amount of Violence Witnessed by Child	0.01	0.07	.02	.91	−.14, .15
Step 2	−				
Amount of Violence Witnessed by Child	0.03	0.08	−.09	.7	−.21, .14
Child Maltreatment	0.34	0.39	.2	.39	−.45, 1.13
Step 3	−				
Amount of Violence Witnessed by Child	0.02	−0.06	−.05	.76	−.15, .11
Child Maltreatment	0.12	0.3	.07	.69	−.49, .73
Mother's PTSS (PCL Total)	0.3	0.06	.67	.001	.16, .43

Note: $R^2 = .000$ for Step 1; $\Delta R^2 = .028$ for Step 2; $\Delta R^2 = .433$ for Step 3 ($p < .001$).

TABLE 3. Hierarchical regression analysis for variables predicting children's total CBCL score

Variable	B	SE B	β	p	95% CI
Step 1					
Child Gender	20.08	9.89	.36	.05	−20, 40.37
Step 2					
Child Gender	15.65	9.84	.28	.12	−4.57, 35.87
Amount of Violence Witnessed by Child	0.41	0.233	.32	.09	−.07, .89
Step 3					
Child Gender	16.89	10.73	.31	.13	−5.20, 38.99
Amount of Violence Witnessed by Child	0.46	0.28	.35	.11	−.11, 1.03
Child Maltreatment	−0.44	1.36	−.07	.75	−3.23, 2.36
Step 4					
Child Gender	19.45	8.03	.35	.02	2.87, 36.03
Amount of Violence Witnessed by Child	0.49	0.21	.38	.03	.07, .92
Child Maltreatment	−1.27	1.03	−.21	.23	−3.39, .86
Mother's PTSS (PCL Total)	0.98	0.22	.61	.001	.54, 1.42

Note: R^2 = .133 for Step 1 (p = .05); ΔR^2 = .094 for Step 2; ΔR^2 = .003 for Step 3; ΔR^2 = .358 for Step 4 (p < .001).

p = .05. The extent of the children's witnessing of violence was added in the second step and was not a significant predictor. The child's own maltreatment score was entered in the third step and was also not a significant predictor. Finally, mother's PTSS score was added in the fourth step and accounted for a significant change in variance, R^2 *change* = .358, β = .609, p < .001; however, this finding should be interpreted with caution. The 95% confidence interval for B for the variable PCL total encompassed the value 1.0, and is thus beyond the scope of this study to identify specifically whether mothers' PTSS contributes to an increase in CBCL scores or a decrease in CBCL scores among children for this sample.

DISCUSSION

Results indicate that a mother's PTSS as a result of her IPV predicted children's emotional functioning, as reported by the mother, after accounting for the extent of the child's witnessing the IPV or the child's own history of maltreatment. Interestingly, neither maltreatment nor extent of witnessing of violence predicted emotion regulation difficulties. These results suggest that a mother's PTSS play a critical role in the child's emotional development, and that the mother's psychological health may in fact influence her child's development more than the child's actual exposure to violence.

This study extends previous researchers' work examining the relationship between maternal PTSD and child behavior (Lieberman et al., 2005) by focusing on emotional functioning outcomes in children of battered women with PTSD. Results suggest that children of mothers with PTSS (including feelings of detachment and estrangement, emotional numbness, and emotion dysregulation) are more emotionally negative and labile. This finding is particularly concerning considering that emotional dysregulation in children can lead to problems in interpersonal relationships, academic problems, and difficulties coping with their environment (Eisenberg et al., 1995; Fabes et al., 1999), putting children at long term developmental risk even after they have been removed from the violent family environment.

One possible explanation for these results is that mothers experiencing posttraumatic stress may not be effective models in how to manage or regulate emotions. Furthermore, a mother's ability to express and feel emotion is a powerful factor in her ability to form a close bond with her child, and this ability is often impaired in PTSD. Finally, if a mother's PTSS are inhibiting her child's ability to have an emotionally satisfying relationship with her, the child may experience more negative emotions and have a more distressing emotional life.

An alternative explanation for these results may be that children of mothers with PTSS show more emotional negativity and lability as a result of acting out in a way that elicits more attention from an emotionally detached mother. A child of such a mother may express more extreme fluctuations of emotion so as to require the mother to intervene and attend to the child's emotion, as these mothers may not be responsive to more subtle emotional expressions in their children if they are themselves numb to emotion.

A final possibility, and a limitation of the design of the study, is that mothers who have PTSS may rate their children as emotionally negative and labile when the children's emotional regulation is actually within a normal range. As this study used a mother's report of children's emotional regulation, it is unknown how well these reports indicate children's actual emotional functioning, as opposed to a mother's subjective view of her child's emotional functioning. Mothers who are emotionally numb or have affect dysregulation may have difficulty understanding or tolerating the expression of emotions in others. It is possible that these mothers may find any emotional expressivity from their children overwhelming, and therefore may be over-pathologizing their children's emotional functioning.

The study's heavy reliance on self and other-report measures represents a major limitation of the study, as they do not necessarily assess how participants and their children actually behave but instead how participants choose to report the behavior. Maternal reports may misrepresent children's emotional problems as a result of mothers' own desire for help, degree of defensiveness, and psychological distress (Hughes, 1988). Several studies have shown that maternal distress can impact mothers' rating of their children's behavior on the CBCL and other measures, with some studies finding that distressed mothers evaluate their children more negatively than they might otherwise (Breslau, Davis, & Prabucki, 1988; Dix, 1991; Forehand, McCombs, & Brody, 1987; Jouriles & Thompson, 1993; Richters, 1992). In contrast, there is some evidence in the literature that mothers may underreport children's behavioral symptomatology. For example, in their study of discrepancies between parental and adolescent reporting of behavior on the CBCL, Seiffge-Krenke and Kollmar (1998) found that mothers underreported their children's internalizing symptoms in comparison to the children's own report. In addition, research with battered women suggests that mothers' preoccupation with her safety during a violent relationship may divert her attention from her child, leading her to overlook or minimize the emotional impact of the child's exposure to violence (Peled & Edleson, 1992). In Chemtob and Carlson's (2004) study, mothers with PTSD were more likely to underestimate distress in their children. In addition, 91% of the mothers with PTSD had not obtained psychiatric services for their children, compared to 46% of the mothers without PTSD.

Another limitation of the study is its small sample size, which limits the stability of these results and the ability to directly test which aspects of PTSD are related to children's adjustment. Future research should attempt to replicate these findings with a larger sample and examine the unique roles of PTSD symptom clusters on parenting and children's adjustment. In addition, research should utilize children's reports of their own functioning, as well as teacher reports of children's functioning to eliminate single informant bias resulting from maternal reports, with additional assessment around how the children experience their mothers' emotional functioning. Observational data would also be a useful addition to this research. In particular, observing the quality of the mother-child interaction and the emotional processes occurring during this interaction would shed some light on the mechanisms by which a mother's PTSS impede her child's emotional functioning.

Given the strong association between mothers' PTSS and the children's emotional development, interventions should focus on treating the mother's PTSS. Many interventions for IPV focus on removing the mother from the violent environment and dealing with the immediate aftereffects of the violent relationship. However, PTSS can exist long after the abuse has ended, and the results of this study suggest that interventions that target these symptoms could have positive implications for children. Cognitive behavior therapies show the most empirical support for treating PTSD (Foa & Meadows, 1997), and cognitive trauma therapy for battered women (CTT-BW; Kubany et al., 2004), which includes PTSD education, stress management, exposure, self-monitoring of negative self-talk, and modules on guilt, self-advocacy, and assertiveness is particularly effective. In addition to treating PTSD symptoms, interventions that target improving parent-child interactions are needed. There is increasing empirical support for the view that therapies targeting the parent-child relationship improve outcomes for children exposed to community violence (Laor, Wolmer, & Cohen, 2001; Linares et al., 2001). Treatments directed at developing affect management skills in both the mothers and their children, such as dialectical behavioral therapy (Linehan, 1993), might be particularly helpful in improving parent-child interactions.

REFERENCES

Achenbach, T. M. (1991). *Manual for the Child Behavior Checklist/4-18 and 1991 profile.* Burlington, VT: University of Vermont, Department of Psychiatry.

American Psychiatric Association. (1994). *Diagnostic and statistical manual of mental disorders* (4th ed.). Washington, DC: Author.

Astin M. C., Lawrence K. J., & Foy D. W. (1993). Posttraumatic stress disorder among battered women: Risk and resiliency factors. *Violence and Victims, 8,* 17–28.

Astin, M. C., Ogland-Hand, S. M., Coleman, E. M., & Foy, D. S (1995). Posttraumatic stress disorder and childhood abuse in battered women: Comparisons with maritally distressed women. *Journal of Consulting and Clinical Psychology, 63,* 308–312.

Blanchard, E. B., Jones-Alexander, J., Buckley, T. C., & Forneris, C. A. (1996). Psychometric properties of the PTSD Checklist (PCL). *Behavior Research Therapy, 34,* 669–673.

Breslau, N., Davis, G. C., & Prabucki, K. (1988). Depressed mothers as informants in family history research: Are they accurate? *Psychiatry Research, 24,* 345–359.

Cassidy, J. (1994). Emotion regulation: Influences of attachment relationships. *Monographs of the Society for Research in Child Development, 59,* 228–249.

Chemtob, C. M., & Carlson, J. G. (2004). Psychological effects of domestic violence on children and their mothers. *International Journal of Stress Management, 11,* 209–226.

Dix, T. (1991). The affective organization of parenting: Adaptive and maladaptive processes. *psychological Bulletin, 110,* 3–25.

Edelson, J. (1999). Children's witnessing of adult domestic violence. *Journal of Interpersonal Violence, 14*, 839–870.

Eisenberg, N., Fabes, R., Murphy, B., Maszk, P., Smith, M., & Karbon, M. (1995). The role of emotionality and regulation in children's social functioning: A longitudinal study. *Child Development, 66*(5), 1360–1384

Fabes, R. A., Eisenberg, N., Jones, S., Smith, M., Guthrie, I., Poulin, R., et al. (1999). Regulation, emotionality, and preschoolers' socially competent peer interactions. *Child Development, 70*, 432–442.

Fantuzzo, J., & Lindquist, C. (1989). The effects of observing conjugal violence on children: A review and analysis of research methodology. *Journal of Family Violence, 4*, 77–94.

Fantuzzo, J. W., & Mohr, W. K. (1999). Prevalence and effects of child exposure to domestic violence. *Future of Children, 9*(3), 21–32.

Foa, E., & Meadows, E. (1997). Psychosocial treatments for post-traumatic stress disorder: A critical review. *Annual Review of Psychology: A Critical Review, 48*, 449–490.

Forehand, R., McCombs, A., & Brody, G. H. (1987). The relationship between parental depressive mood states and child functioning. *Advances in Behavior Research & Therapy, 9*(1), 1–20.

Harkness, L. L. (1993). Transgenerational transmission of war-related trauma. In J. P. Wilson & B. Raphael (Eds.), *International handbook of traumatic stress syndromes* (pp. 635–643). New York: Plenum.

Hughes, H. M. (1982). Brief intervention with children in a battered women's shelter: A model preventive program. *Family Relations, 31*, 495–502.

Hughes, H. M. (1988). Psychological and behavioral correlates of family violence in child witnesses and victims. *American Journal of Orthopsychiatry, 58*, 77–90.

Jordan, B. K., Marmar, C. R., Fairbank, J. A., Schlenger, W. E., Kulka, R. A., Hough, R. L., et al. (1992). Problems in families of male Vietnam veterans with posttraumatic stress disorder. *Journal of Consulting and Clinical Psychology, 60*, 916–926.

Jouriles, E. N., & Thompson, S. M. (1993). Effects of mood on mothers' evaluations of children's behavior. *Journal of Family Psychology, 6*, 300–307.

Kracke, K., & Hahn, H. (2008). The nature and extent of childhood exposure to violence: What we know, why we don't know more, and why it matters. *Journal of Emotional Abuse, 8*(1/2), 29–49.

Kubany, E., Hill, E., Owens, J., Iannce-Spencer, C., McCaig, M., Tremayne, K., et al. (2004). Cognitive trauma therapy for battered women with PTSD (CTT-BW). *Journal of Consulting and Clinical Psychology, 72*, 3–18.

Laor, N., Wolmer, L., & Cohen, D. (2001). Mothers' functioning and children's symptoms 5 years after a SCUD missile attack. *American Journal of Psychiatry, 159*, 1020–1026.

Lieberman, A. F., Van Horn, P., & Ozer, E. (2005). Preschooler witnesses of marital violence: Predictors and mediators of child behavior problems. *Development and Psychopathology, 17*, 385–396.

Linares, L., Heeren, T., Bronfman, E., Zuckerman, B., Augustyn, M., & Tronick, E. (2001). A mediational model for the impact of exposure to community violence on early child behavior problems. *Child Development, 72*, 639–652.

Linehan, M. M. (1993). *Skills training manual for treating borderline personality disorder.* New York: The Guilford Press.

Margolin, G. (1998). Effects of domestic violence on children. In P. K. Trickett & C. J. Shellenbach (Eds.), *Violence against children in the family and community* (pp. 57–101). Washington, DC: American Psychological Association.

Margolin, G., & Gordis, E. B. (2000). The effects of family and community violence on children. *Annual Review of Psychology, 51,* 445–479.

Peled, E., & Edleson, J. (1992). Multiple perspectives on groupwork with children of battered women. *Violence and Victims, 7,* 327–346.

Pynoos, R. W., & Eth, S. (1985). *Posttraumatic stress disorder in children.* Washington, DC: American Psychiatric Association Press.

Resnick, H., & Acierno, R. (1997). Health impact of interpersonal violence: Medical and mental health outcomes. *Behavioral Medicine, 23,* 53–64.

Richters, J. E. (1992). Depressed mothers as informants about their children: A critical review of the evidence for distortion. *Psychological Bulletin, 112,* 485–499.

Ruscio, A. M., Weathers, F. W., & King, L. A. (2002). Male war-zone veterans' perceived relationships with their children: The importance of emotional numbing. *Journal of Traumatic Stress, 15*(5), 351–357.

Samper, R., Taft, C., King, D., & King, L. (2004). Posttraumatic stress disorder symptoms and parenting satisfaction among a national sample of male Vietnam veterans. *Journal of Traumatic Stress, 17*(4), 311–315.

Saunders, D. G. (1994). Post-traumatic stress symptom profiles of battered women: A comparison of survivors in two settings. *Violence and Victims, 9,* 31–44.

Seiffge-Krenke, I., & Kollmar, F. (1998). Discrepancies between mothers' and fathers' perceptions of sons' and daughters' problem behavior: A longitudinal analysis of parent-adolescent agreement on internalizing and externalizing problem behavior. *Journal of Child Psychology and Psychiatry, 39*(5), 687–697.

Shields, A., & Cicchetti, D. (1997). Emotion regulation among school-age children: The development and validation of a new criterion Q-sort scale. *Developmental Psychology, 33,* 906–916.

Straus, M. (1992). Children as witnesses to marital violence: A risk factor of lifelong problems among a nationally representative sample of American men and women. In D. Schwartz (Ed.), *Children and violence: Report of the twenty-third Ross roundtable on critical approaches to common pediatric problems.* Columbus, OH: Ross Lab.

Straus, M. A. (1979). Measuring intrafamily conflict and violence: The Conflict Tactics Scales. *Journal of Marriage and Family, 41,* 75–88.

Straus, M. A., Hamby, S. L., Boney-McCoy, S., & Sugarman, D. B. (1996). The revised Conflict Tactics Scales (CTS2): Development and preliminary psychometric data. *Journal of Family Issues, 17,* 283–316.

Weathers, F. W., Litz, B. T., Herman, D. S., Huska, J. A., & Keane, T. M. (1993, October). *The PTSD Checklist: Reliability, validity and diagnostic utility.* Paper presented at the annual meeting of the International Society for Traumatic Stress Studies, San Antonio, TX.

Wolfe, D., Jaffe, P., Wilson, S. K., & Zak, L. (1985). Children of battered women: The relation of child behavior to family violence and maternal stress. *Journal of Consulting and Clinical Psychology, 53*(5), 657–665.

The Safe Start Initiative: Building and Disseminating Knowledge to Support Children Exposed to Violence

Kristen Kracke
Elena P. Cohen

Safe Start is a collaborative initiative involving national, state, and local public and private agencies led and coordinated by the U.S. Department of Justice's (DOJs) Office of Juvenile Justice and Delinquency Prevention (OJJDP) with the goal of preventing and reducing the consequences of children's exposure to violence. The impetus for the development of this initiative was the recognition of the need to address children's exposure to violence as a critical prevention strategy for juvenile delinquency and the necessity of developing policy and intervention strategies across sectors and disciplines in the context of the nature, extent, and consequences of children's exposure to violence.

In April 1997, the White House convened the national Early Childhood Development and Learning Conference to discuss strategies to disseminate results of research on brain development to a variety of professionals working with young children. The DOJ was charged with establishing the Safe Start Initiative to help break the cycle of violence for the nation's youngest victims. At the conference, it was recommended that Safe Start provide intensive training and technical assistance nationwide for professionals who come into contact with children who have been exposed to family violence, violence in their community and schools, and abuse or neglect (U.S. Department of Education, 1997).

Subsequently, in 1999, DOJ and the U.S. Department of Health and Human Services (HHS) convened the National Summit on Children Exposed to Violence—Safe from the Start Summit. This summit of practitioners and policymakers was convened to build on their commitment to a common goal, think through the problem of children exposed to violence, and create a framework for a national blueprint for action. Summit participants included professionals from both the public and the private sectors who worked to find common ground across their different professional vocabularies, assumptions about the nature of the problem, and views on the solutions. In the end, this summit transformed a set of key operating principles and concrete steps into a practical action agenda for local, state, and national leaders; professionals across disciplines; communities; and parents, youth, and families to prevent and reduce the impact of children's exposure to violence. These recommendations were described in the National Action Plan (U.S. Department of Justice, 2000). Launched at the Safe from the Start Summit, the Safe Start Initiative was designed in concert with the summit recommendations in the 6 months leading up to the event. It was led by OJJDP in collaboration with other offices in the Office of Justice Programs at DOJ and with HHS.

Several considerations framed the design of the initiative. Exposure to violence has become viewed as a public health issue because of its negative impact on the short- and long-term health and well-being of children and communities. Using this public health approach, Safe Start called for a continuum of services moving from prevention, through early intervention, treatment, and crisis response and provided the framework for research and interventions that draws on the insights and strategies of diverse disciplines. In addition, because information dissemination is a critical element of the public health mission, Safe Start, since its beginning, has acknowledged the importance of raising awareness about the problem and the solutions and broadening the knowledge base (Mercy, 1993).

At the time Safe Start was launched, there was a growing research consensus stating the detrimental effects of all types of exposure to violence on children. Available prevalence data at the time broadly estimated that between 3.3 million and 10 million children witnessed domestic violence each year in the United States (Carlson, 1984; Straus, 1991), but estimates combining all types of exposure to violence were not available. Practitioners working in different systems were beginning to design interventions specific to their work settings. These interventions had varying degrees of evaluation, but in general, there was limited evidence to support the effectiveness of the interventions and no national repository of the information for easy access (U.S. DOJ, 2000).

Concurrently, to respond to the growing consensus that the human service system providing services to the nation's most vulnerable families was often ineffective and to break down discrete, single-discipline "silos," human service practitioners, policymakers, and administrators were partnering to find new strategies for implementing service integration efforts. These efforts included joint policies and memorandums of understanding for shared service delivery, co-location of services, shared resources, inclusion of families in system development, cross-system training, and broad-based community inclusion with specific roles and responsibilities (Melaville & Blank, 1993). In June 1999, OJJDP developed the Safe Start Initiative to prevent and reduce the impact of exposure to child maltreatment, domestic violence, and community violence on children and their families.

THE SAFE START INITIATIVE

Since its inception and throughout the process of implementation, the Safe Start Initiative has aimed to broaden the "silo-ed" definitions of exposure to violence. It has done this by building public and professional awareness of the issues to create a comprehensive service delivery system encompassing prevention, early intervention, treatment, and response and to improve the access to, delivery of, and quality of services both for children at high risk of being exposed to violence and for those who have already been exposed.

Theoretical Foundation

Safe Start is rooted in developmental and systems theories. An ecological theory and transactional model of behavior approaches behavior as multi-determined and driven largely by the relationships that individuals have with other systems with which they interact. Ecological theory views developing children and their families as embedded in multiple systems that have direct and indirect influences on their behavior and these influences are reciprocal and bi-directional. The transactional approach asserts that each child's development phase is impacted not only by the current environmental factors but also by past experiences in the context of the earlier stages of development (Brofenbrenner, 1979; Dawes & Donald, 2000; Edmond, Fitzgerald, & Kracke, 2005).

Figure 1 illustrates the complex range of environmental and developmental risks and protective factors within the child, relationship context (family), immediate social context (community), and the larger society that may prevent or increase the negative impacts of exposure to violence. For example, just as the intensity of a single event may determine a

FIGURE 1. The Interplay of the Ecological and Transactional Models on Development.

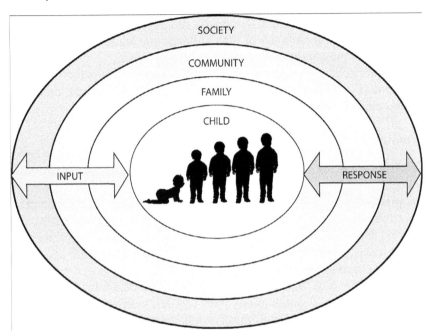

child's reaction to that event, so does the child's developmental stage, chronicity of the exposure, and current environment.

Core Principles

Safe Start participants, partners, and a multidisciplinary group of professionals and practitioners applied this theoretical framework to what was known about the prevalence, consequences, and treatment of exposure to violence. They developed and applied the following principles to guide the Safe Start work of creating a continuum of care for children exposed to violence:

- The impact of children's exposure to violence depends on risk and resiliency factors internal to the child and in the family, community, and larger society.
- Policies and practices for children exposed to violence need to balance *innovation* with *efficacy*.

- It is essential to increase both *awareness* about children exposed to violence and *identification* of children exposed to violence in all systems supporting and serving families.
- Interventions for families living with domestic violence *must* ensure the safety and well-being of both children and adults at all points of entry into the continuum of care.
- All practices and supports in the continuum of care for children exposed to violence must be developmentally appropriate, tailored, and evidence-based.

Framework

To implement its core principles and meet its goals, Safe Start was designed as a comprehensive national framework. This framework supports practice innovation through Safe Start communities funded competitively through OJJDP, expands the knowledge base of evidence-based practices, and creates and coordinates a national repository of resources to support local and national practice innovations to address the needs of children exposed to violence.

Phase I of the Safe Start Initiative engaged "Demonstration Site" communities in creating a continuum of care. The development of strategies in this continuum of care was built mostly on literature available on the negative impacts of exposure, particularly among young children. Phase II, the Safe Start Promising Approaches, draws on the findings, innovations, and experiences of the demonstration sites along with continued advancements in evidence-based practices in the exposure-to-violence field. These sites are engaged in a rigorous quasi-experimental evaluation that will inform Phase III. Phase III will replicate findings and experiences of the promising approaches sites to further evaluate and confirm results. Phase IV will broadly infuse the effective interventions and practices by seeding the practice knowledge in as many sites as possible; this final phase will continue as the knowledge transfer is infused and practices are strengthened and expanded to effectively prevent and reduce the impact of children's exposure to violence. Figure 2 illustrates the phased implementation framework.

SAFE START COMPONENTS

The core components that support this framework and constitute the overall Safe Start Initiative include research and evaluation; training and

FIGURE 2. Safe Start National Framework.

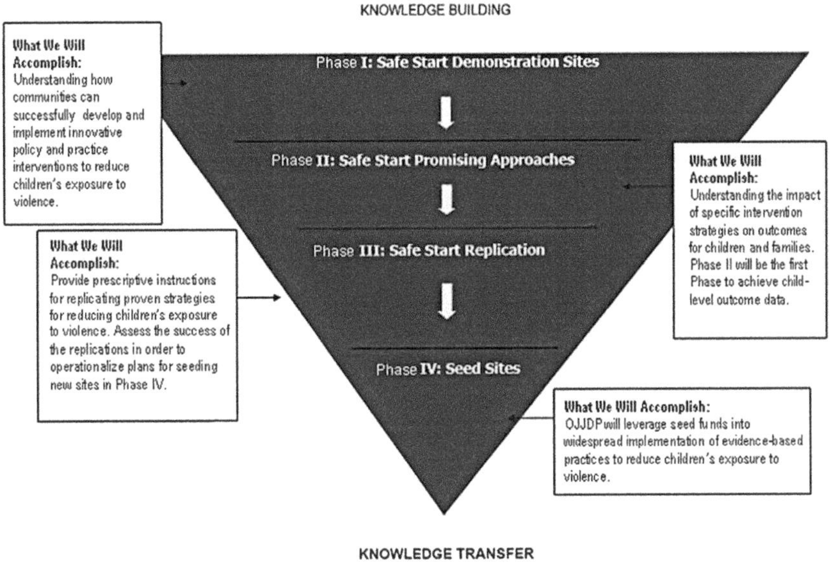

KNOWLEDGE BUILDING

What We Will Accomplish:
Understanding how communities can successfully develop and implement innovative policy and practice interventions to reduce children's exposure to violence.

Phase I: Safe Start Demonstration Sites

Phase II: Safe Start Promising Approaches

What We Will Accomplish:
Understanding the impact of specific intervention strategies on outcomes for children and families. Phase II will be the first Phase to achieve child-level outcome data.

What We Will Accomplish:
Provide prescriptive instructions for replicating proven strategies for reducing children's exposure to violence. Assess the success of the replications in order to operationalize plans for seeding new sites in Phase IV.

Phase III: Safe Start Replication

Phase IV: Seed Sites

What We Will Accomplish:
OJJDP will leverage seed funds into widespread implementation of evidence-based practices to reduce children's exposure to violence.

KNOWLEDGE TRANSFER

technical assistance, resource development, and dissemination of information; partnerships and alliances; and practice innovation. These components are supported by a cadre of national and local organizations and are discussed below.

Research and Evaluation

The research and evaluation component consists of three elements: (a) a national incidence and prevalence study on children exposed to violence, (b) the national evaluation of the Safe Start demonstration sites, and (c) the national evaluation of the promising approaches sites. The National Study on Children Exposed to Violence is under development at the University of New Hampshire's Crimes Against Children Research Center. This national study builds on the center's previous and ongoing work with the Juvenile Victimization Questionnaire (Finkelhor, Ormrod, Turner, & Hamby, 2005). The study is supported and coordinated by OJJDP under the Safe Start Initiative to provide robust national numbers on children's exposure to violence, using a broad definition of exposure that incorporates multiple events and types of exposure. Currently in the design phase, this comprehensive assessment will examine a variety of potential predictors and outcomes of children's exposure to violence and will likely use a randomized telephone survey to obtain a target sample of 4,000–6,000 children between ages 2 and 17 (Finkelhor, Ormrod, & Turner, 2007).

Evaluation of the Safe Start communities has been conducted under the individual phases of practice development. The Association for the Study and Development of Community (ASDC) conducted the national evaluation for the demonstration sites under Phase I, and the RAND Corporation is conducting the national evaluation of the promising approaches sites. The design elements for each evaluation are described below under the demonstration sites and promising approaches sites sections.

Training and Technical Assistance, Resource Development, and Dissemination of Information

Two national resource centers—working closely with each other and with local communities—have developed tools and other materials relevant to children's exposure to violence in different settings. These resources are available to the public through the Internet and are disseminated to a broad range of target audiences, including practitioners in all areas and disciplines, parents, administrators, policymakers, and the general public, with the goal of translating the current knowledge base into tools and practical briefs.

The National Center on Children Exposed to Violence (NCCEV) at the Yale Child Study Center grew from the expertise of the Child Development-Community Policing (CD-CP) model, one of the foremost models of acute response mental health–law enforcement partnerships. Through this specialized content expertise, the NCCEV provided intensive training and technical assistance support to the Safe Start demonstration sites in Phase I and has served to increase the capacity of individuals and communities to reduce the incidence and impact of violence on children and families through training and awareness building particularly in the area of mental health involvement.

The Safe Start Center is the national resource center designed to support the Safe Start Initiative as well as build and disseminate the knowledge gained through the work of the initiative. This support includes working with national partners and a multidisciplinary group of experts to provide training and technical assistance to the 15 promising approaches pilot sites and resource development and information dissemination on Safe Start and other national advancements in the field of exposure to violence. The Safe Start Center provides training and technical assistance to the 26 Safe Start communities and to practitioners and communities across the country through consultation, intensive onsite technical support, training, and maintenance of a national database of consultants with specific technical and content expertise. The center recruits additional expert consultants and provides both matching services and effectiveness assessments. The center convenes national and regional Safe Start meetings and addresses other related topics to foster a learning community and ensure the efficient sharing of knowledge and skills among grantees, national partners, and those in the field.

Partnerships and Alliances

Throughout the implementation of Safe Start, OJJDP and the initiative team, comprising RAND, ASDC, Safe Start Center, Safe Start sites, and NCCEV, have collaborated formally and informally with a wide range of national and local partners with a strong commitment to addressing the exposure to violence issue. These collaborations have enhanced knowledge, skills, and abilities to address the impact of exposure to violence on young children and their families and to disseminate information on innovations and promising practices. National partners include Zero to Three; the Family Violence Prevention Fund; the Child Witness to Violence Project; the Institute for Community Peace; the American Psychological Association; the National Council of Juvenile and Family Court Judges; the Early Trauma Treatment Network; the California State Attorney General's Office; the Institute of Violence, Abuse, and Trauma at Alliant International University; the National Civic League; the Institute for Educational Leadership; and others.

Practice Innovation: The Safe Start Communities

Demonstration Sites

Eleven Safe Start demonstration sites received funding during Phase I: Baltimore, MD; Bridgeport, CT; Chatham County, NC; Chicago, IL; Pinellas County, FL; Pueblo of Zuni, NM; Rochester, NY; San Francisco, CA; Sitka Tribe of Alaska; Spokane, WA; and Washington County, ME.

Safe Start demonstration sites improved the system of care for young children exposed to violence and their families by implementing a balanced, comprehensive approach across a full continuum of prevention, intervention, treatment, and response. These improvements focused on five domains of system change: (a) development of policies, procedures, and protocols; (b) service integration activities; (c) resource development, identification, and reallocation; (d) expanded and enhanced programming; and (e) community action and awareness. To ensure the sustainability of these system improvement strategies, sites implemented strategies across three levels of the service delivery system: (a) across different agencies, (b) within each organization (supervisors and midlevel managers), and (c) at the point of service delivery (frontline staff, families, and children).

Each of the 11 demonstration communities implemented a tailored, locally driven approach using strategies based on the service strengths, gaps, needs, and cultural and geographic distinctions of the community and its service delivery system. Several strategies were developed to address challenges associated with existing service delivery systems and to build on the promising new directions for prevention, intervention, and treatment that were emerging in the field.

Some of the promising practices implemented are described:

- Improving identification, screening, and referral strategies and practices. For example, Spokane, WA, added a question to the 911 protocol regarding the presence of children when a domestic violence call is received. In Bridgeport, CT, a protocol was developed and used by child protection workers to screen families for domestic violence and refer them to appropriate services.
- Improving responses by integrating services and enhancing programming. For example, in Washington County, ME, a formal review process for cross-disciplinary professional providers was developed to share information about families, conduct joint service planning, and reduce the isolation of individual service providers. Chatham, NC, provided intensive home-based therapy services in English and Spanish.
- Engaging and retaining families in voluntary services. For example, Spokane, WA, developed a protocol for the police to get verbal permission from the family to call the child outreach team as a voluntary support service.
- Increasing cultural competence. For example, San Francisco, CA, translated all its forms into Spanish and Chinese, used ethnic media and organizations to reach the Spanish- and Chinese-speaking communities, and engaged same-gender families. Pueblo Zuni, NM, focused on the use of the Zuni language and wove in Safe Start messages to increase awareness of traditions and cultural practices.

- Raising community awareness. For example, Pinellas County, FL, and Rochester, NY, developed social marketing and public educational campaigns that effectively increased the willingness of community members to respond to children's exposure to violence.

To implement these new policies and programs, the demonstration sites established collaborative partnerships among service providers in the fields of early childhood/development, health, mental health, family support and strengthening, domestic violence, substance abuse prevention and treatment, crisis intervention, child welfare, law enforcement, courts, and legal services. In addition, the demonstration sites engaged community agencies, systems, and leaders in raising awareness about issues related to children's exposure to violence and in identifying, developing, and reallocating resources to promote the Safe Start vision (Association for the Study and Development of Community, 2006).

Evaluation of the Safe Start demonstration sites. To develop a better understanding of how communities can successfully minimize the negative consequences of exposure to violence by implementing a comprehensive system of care, ASDC conducted a comprehensive evaluation with the following design components: (a) a cross-site analysis, (b) a process evaluation, (c) case studies of each of the 11 sites, and (d) six local child-level outcome studies. The ASDC collected and reported data on the 11 initiatives that described their implementation process and the clients served and highlighted some of the sites' promising practices (ASDC, 2005a).

The ASDC partnered with local evaluators to develop case studies that used a common framework and common data elements for cross-site analysis and knowledge development. In addition, ASDC enhanced the capacity of sites to measure and collect data, and as a result, all demonstration sites increased their ability to use information for improving the quality of project implementation and outcomes (ASDC, 2005b). This capacity-building work supported the iterative planning process embedded in the design and has helped increase success in sustaining the initiative in each site now that direct federal funding has ended.

Accomplishments of the Safe Start demonstration sites. The accomplishments of the demonstration sites include the following (ASDC, 2006):

- Increased public awareness of exposure to violence in the community. Several sites conducted award-winning social marketing and public education campaigns.

- New working relationships among sectors based on the issue of exposure to violence, including sharing case information and management among collaborative providers.
- Comprehensive and coordinated systems of care to respond to the needs of children and their families. For example, some sites were successful at co-locating services for children exposed to violence in different agencies and systems.
- Institutionalized training to expand the knowledge and skills of service providers and their organizations.
- Changes in state policies to respond to children exposed to violence and their families.
- Increased capacity to adapt interventions to reduce the impact of exposure to violence on children. For example, several sites adapted and implemented mental health–law enforcement partnerships for acute response based on the CD-CP model.

Hyde, Lamb, and Chavis (2008, this issue) provide full descriptions of the Safe Start demonstration sites' cross-site and case study evaluation and promising practices.

Promising Approaches Sites

The overall vision and goals for Phase II remain the same as those for Phase I; however, the main objective of the Safe Start promising approaches communities is to pilot test and measure the effectiveness of key evidence-based intervention strategies drawn from the emergent children exposed to violence literature, with the informed premise that these evidence-based strategies will prevent and reduce the negative impact of exposure to violence. Fifteen communities in the following cities are being supported with federal funding from 2000 to 2009: Bronx, NY; Chelsea, MA; Dallas, TX; Dayton, OH; Erie, PA; Kalamazoo, MI; Miami, FL; New York City, NY; Oakland, CA; Pompano, FL; Portland, OR; Providence, RI; Toledo, OH; San Diego, CA; and San Mateo, CA. These communities are expanding partnerships among service providers in areas such as early childhood education/development, health, mental health, child welfare, family support, domestic violence/crisis intervention, law enforcement, the courts, and legal services. Safe Start integrates and sometimes expands interventions that have empirical support and demonstrate promising or recommended practices. For example, different psychotherapeutic interventions involve both the parent caregiver and the child or infant (Adams, Osofsky, Hammer, & Graham, 2003; Cohen, Mannarino, Berliner, & Deblinger, 2000; Herschell, Calzada, Eyberg, & McNeil, 2002; Jentoft-Kinniburgh & Blaustein, nd; Lieberman & Van Horn, 2005; Taylor, Gilbert, Mann, & Ryan, 2005; Toth, Maughan, Manly, Spagnola, & Cichetti, 2002; Zero to Three, 2000); medical home (recommended by the American Academy of Pediatrics, 2002); home visitations (Mihalic, Fagan, Irwin, Ballard, & Elliott, 2004); child advocacy centers (Jones, nd); specialized curricula (University of Missouri-St. Louis, 2006); motivational interviewing (Hettema, Steele, & Miller, 2005); family support (Jouriles, McDonald, Spiller, Norwood, & Swank, 2001); cultural competence (Blase & Fixsen, 2003); service coordination (Soler, 1992); integrated mental health/case management (Utah State University, 2005); domestic violence–child welfare collaborations (Schechter & Edleson, 1999); support services for kinship care providers (Schmidt, 2005); family-centered services (University of Virginia, Richmond, 2002); partnerships with dependency courts (Lederman, Osofsky, & Katz, 2001); and the Kids Club intervention (Graham-Bermann, 1997).

Evaluation of the promising approaches sites. The RAND Corporation is conducting a comprehensive evaluation to assess the effectiveness of the interventions at the child level and to examine the variability in the intervention effects, identifying plausible reasons for the variability. On completion of the evaluation study, RAND, OJJDP, and the Safe Start communities will answer the following research questions: Is the Safe Start intervention associated with positive outcomes for children? What programmatic elements represent best practices? How are the program costs associated with the observed outcomes? What are the underlying protective processes involved in developing resiliency over time?

The evaluation design is composed of the following elements: (a) a quasi-experimental comparison study, (b) process evaluation, and (c) a training evaluation component. The comparison study will enable RAND to collect longitudinal, individual-level data and analyze the individual-level outcomes within sites, across clusters of sites with similar intervention characteristics, and across all sites. The process evaluation will collect data from multiple sources and describe key features of each site and its intervention. The training evaluation will collect data related to staff and community partners involved in the intervention and will assess the impact of training on knowledge, attitudes, and practice. Preliminary findings for the 15 promising approaches sites are expected in 2010.

The implementation of the Safe Start Initiative is showing that pathways exist to prevent and reduce the negative impacts of children's exposure to violence. The future challenge will be to increase the knowledge base, to translate the knowledge into practice, and to disseminate the information to those working with children and families across the country.

REFLECTING FORWARD

When Safe Start was initially developed, the field of children's exposure to violence was a mere 10 years old and emerging (Edleson, 2004; Kracke, 2005). During the last 7 years of the initiative's implementation, the field has improved significantly in building public and professional awareness of the issues as well as in reaching across disciplines and system entry points to increase informed services, training, and cross-training and to build an emergent evidence base for practice. Definitional issues continue to make it difficult to get a precise figure on the number of children exposed to violence in their homes, schools, and community (see Kracke & Hahn, 2008, this issue). However, clear indicators from the Safe Start Initiative and other research efforts show that the magnitude and impact of violence is a substantial and serious global problem. It occurs in every country in the world in a variety of forms and settings and is often deeply rooted in cultural, economic, and social practices (Pinheiro, 2006; see Chamberlain (2008, this issue) and Willmon-Haque and Bigfoot (2008, this issue) for further discussion on cultural issues).

Compelling evidence from neuroscience about the influence of early relationships and experience on the architecture of the brain (Schonkoff & Phillips, 2000) and cognitive, social, and emotional development of the child has led to the increase of policy and practice attention on infants and toddlers. Encouraged by positive research findings from Early Head Start and other programs, a number of states and communities are investing in programs to promote healthy relationships and prevent problems, particularly in low-income and caregiver families. However, children can suffer from what scientists call "toxic stress" from a variety of environmental conditions such as an inconsistent caregiver, neglect, or stress without violence. Children who are exposed to violence in the home or the community may need specialized and intensive supports to put them back on the path to healthy development (Knitzer & Cohen, 2007; National Scientific Council on the Developing Child, 2006).

Concurrently, an emerging body of social science research indicates that, as a group, children exposed to violence have significantly higher rates of behavioral and emotional problems and academic failures (Edleson, 1999). The research evidence on children's exposure to violence consistently indicates that the timing, frequency, and intensity of adverse experiences are associated with a magnitude of negative developmental outcomes (McAlister Groves, 2002). Furthermore, in the case of prolonged exposure to violence, there are indications that the disruption of nervous and immune systems can lead to social, emotional, and cognitive impairments, as well as behaviors that cause disease, injury, and social problems (Feerick & Silverman, 2006).

In the clinical field, data to support the effectiveness of different strategies and protocols in a broad array of environments are being collected across the country. Critical components of successful interventions include a developmental perspective that engages the child's and family's ecological contexts and service systems to screen for, provide early intervention for, and respond to the treatment needs of children. In addition, it has become evident that effectiveness is bolstered when treatment is offered in a range of settings, such as homes, early care and education programs, and schools, incorporating collaboration with health, police, legal, child welfare, and other systems (Lieberman & DiMartino, 2005).

Along with the Safe Start communities, a number of coordinated efforts during the last decade—for example, the Green Book Initiative communities, the National Child Traumatic Stress Network, the Safe and Bright Futures projects, the Domestic Violence Initiative for Child Protective Services at the Massachusetts Department of Social Services, the CD-CP projects, the Miami Model Dependency Court Safe Start, the Child Witness to Violence Project at Boston Medical Center, the Violence Intervention Program at Louisiana State University, and the Child Trauma Research Project at San Francisco General Hospital—are encouraging systems and communities to move beyond individual agencies to respond to the effects of violence on children in a more collaborative, comprehensive way.

Across neurological, social, clinical, and other applied sciences, it has become apparent that achieving a comprehensive system of response to children exposed to violence will require sufficient resources, increased awareness of the problem, new and enhanced policies, an array of intervention approaches, and the development of an agreed-on national research agenda that defines exposure to violence broadly and inclusively. With allocation of adequate resources, policies and programs can address immediate factors such as the development of nurturing environments that facilitate parent–child attachment, support families, and challenge social norms that condone violence (Knitzer & Lefkowitz, 2006). Raising the awareness about the harmful effects of exposure to violence is necessary not only for the general public but also to enhance the capacity of those who work with and for children and families. Development of tools, training, supervision, and other staff supports and resources will build capacity not only to provide children exposed to violence and their families with high-quality effective programs but also to identify these children early and, therefore, provide them with an opportunity to successfully alter their paths. This capacity-building must occur across all disciplines and service sectors. Across these same sectors, policies and procedures must be enhanced and expanded to ensure that children at risk are identified early and referred to appropriate service entities. These services must be accessible, affordable, and provided in a culturally respectful manner. Lastly, developing a consensus on a national research agenda on exposure to violence continues to be critical for building knowledge and improving practices. Understanding the magnitude of the problem of children's exposure to violence through a broad and inclusive lens is a critical next step.

As a strategic national initiative, Safe Start builds toward these long-term goals and serves to move the field forward by working together with national and local partners. Safe Start contributes a coordinated infusion of resources focusing on the problem of children exposed to violence, which increases the capacity of practitioners, administrators, policymakers, and researchers in the public and private sectors to effectively prevent and reduce the impact of exposure to violence. The strategic work and the leadership of the Safe Start partnerships will move the field from knowledge-building to a point of knowledge-transfer. A decade from now Safe Start will provide policymakers with a specific national direction guided by evidence of which interventions make a difference and the long-term results of these investments in both science and practice. Researchers, practitioners in different disciplines, and families will have a set of resources and tools to develop solid cross-sector practice and training as well as a shared understanding of the incidence and prevalence of exposure to violence and its impact on the child, the family, and the community.

REFERENCES

Adams, S., Osofsky, J., Hammer, J. H., & Graham, M. (2003). *Program evaluation: Florida Infant & Mental Health Pilot Project Year 3 Final Report: July 1, 2000 to June 25, 2003*. Tallahassee, FL: Florida State University, Center for Prevention & Early Intervention Policy.

American Academy of Pediatrics. (2002). *Policy statement: Medical home.* Retrieved February 14, 2007, http://aappolicy.aappublications.org/cgi/reprint/pediatrics;110/1/184.pdf.

Association for the Study and Development of Community. (2005a). *National evaluation of the Safe Start demonstration: Cross-site evaluation.* Gaithersburg, MD: Author. Retrieved February 2, 2007, http://www.safestartcenter.org

Association for the Study and Development of Community. (2005b). *National evaluation of the Safe Start demonstration: Case studies of demonstration sites.* Gaithersburg, MD: Author. Retrieved February 2, 2007, http://www.safestartcenter.org

Association for the Study and Development of Community. (2006). *Promising practices of Safe Start demonstration project sites: 1995.* Gaithersburg, MD: Author. Retrieved February 2, 2007, http://www.safestartcenter.org

Blase, K., & Fixsen, D. (2003). *National implementation research network consensus statement on evidence-based programs and cultural competence.* Tampa, FL: Louis de la Parte Florida Mental Health Institute.

Brofenbrenner, U. (1979). *The ecology of human development: Experiments by nature and design.* Cambridge, MA: Harvard University Press.

Carlson, B. E. (1984). Children's observations of interpersonal violence. In A. Roberts (Ed.), *Battered women and their families* (pp. 147–167). New York: Springer.

Chamberlain, L. (2008). Ten lessons learned in Alaska: Home visitation and intimate partner violence. *Journal of Emotional Abuse, 8*(1/2), 205–216.

Cohen, J., Mannarino, A., Berliner, L., & Deblinger, J. (2000). Trauma-focused cognitive behavioral therapy for children and adolescents: An empirical update. *Journal of Interpersonal Violence, 15*(11), 1202–1223.

Dawes, A., & Donald, D. (2000). Improving children's chances: Developmental theory and effective interventions in community contexts. In D. Donald, A. Dawes, & J. Louw (Eds.), *Addressing childhood adversity* (pp. 1–25). Cape Town, South Africa: David Philip.

Edleson, J. (2004). Should childhood exposure to adult domestic violence be defined as child maltreatment under the law? In P. G. Jaffe, L. L. Baker, & A. J. Cunningham (Eds.), *Protecting children from domestic violence: Strategies for community intervention* (pp. 8–29). New York: Guilford Press.

Edleson, J. L. (1999). Children's witnessing of adult domestic violence. *Journal of Interpersonal Violence, 14*(8), 39–70.

Edmond, Y., Fitzgerald, M., & Kracke, K. (2005). *Incidence and prevalence of children exposed to violence: A research review.* Unpublished manuscript.

Feerick, M., & Silverman, G. G. (2006). *Children exposed to violence.* Baltimore, MD: Paul Brooks Publishing.

Finkelhor, D., Ormrod, R., & Turner H. (2007). Poly-victimization: A neglected component in child victimization. *Child Abuse and Neglect, 31*, 7–26.

Finkelhor, D., Ormrod, R., Turner, H., & Hamby, S. L. (2005). The victimization of children and youth: A comprehensive, national survey. *Child Maltreatment, 10*, 5–25.

Graham-Bermann, S. (1997). *The Kids Club: Intervention with groups of children in families with domestic violence.* Unpublished manuscript, University of Michigan, Ann Arbor.

Herschell, A. D., Calzada, E. J., Eyberg, S. M., & McNeil, C. B. (2002). Research on parent-child interaction therapy: Past and future. *Cognitive and Behavioral Practice, 9,* 9–16.

Hettema, J., Steele, J., & Miller, W. R. (2005). A meta-analysis of research on motivational interviewing treatment effectiveness (MARMITE). *Annual Review of Clinical Psychology 1,* 91–111.

Hyde, M. M., Lamb, Y. H., & Chavis, D. (2008). Safe Start: Promising practices from the evaluation of the demonstration project Association for the Study and Development of Community. *Journal of Emotional Abuse, 8*(1/2), 175–186.

Jentoft-Kinniburgh, K., & Blaustein, M. (nd). *Attachment, self-regulation, and competence (ARC): A common-sense framework for intervention with complexly traumatized youth.* Unpublished report.

Jones, L. (nd). *Multi-site evaluation of child advocacy centers.* Retrieved February 8, 2007, from University of New Hampshire, Durham, Crimes Against Children Research Center website: http://www.unh.edu/ccrc/multi-site_evaluation_children.html

Jouriles, E., McDonald, R., Spiller, L., Norwood, W., & Swank, P. (2001). Reducing conduct problems among children of battered women. *Journal of Consulting & Clinical Psychology, 69,* 774–785.

Knitzer, J., & Cohen E. (2007). Promoting resilience in young children and families at the highest risk: The challenge for early childhood mental health. In D. Perry, R. Kaufman, & J. Knitzer (Eds.), *Social & emotional health in early childhood: Building bridges between services & systems* (pp. 335–359). Baltimore, MD: Brookes.

Knitzer, J., & Lefkowitz, J. (2006). *Helping the most vulnerable children and their families.* New York: National Center for Children in Poverty.

Kracke, K. (2005, September). Reflecting forward. *Safe Start Newsletter, 4,* 1–2.

Kracke, K., & Hahn, H. (2008). The nature and extent of childhood exposure to violence: What we know, why we don't *know more, and why* it matters. *Journal of Emotional Abuse, 8*(1/2), 29–49.

Lederman, C., Osofsky, J., & Katz, L. (2001). When the bough breaks the cradle will fall: Promoting the health and well-being of infants and toddlers in juvenile court. *Juvenile and Family Court Journal, 52*(4), 4–8.

Lieberman, A., & DiMartino, R. (Eds.). (2005). *Johnson & Johnson Pediatric Series, 6. Interventions for children exposed to violence.* Key Biscayne, FL: Johnson & Johnson, Inc.

Lieberman, A. F., & Van Horn, P. (2005). *Don't hit my mommy! A manual for child–parent psychotherapy with young witnesses of family violence.* Washington, DC: Zero to Three Press.

McAlister Groves, B. (2002). *Children who see too much.* Boston, MA: Beacon Press.

Melaville, A. I., & Blank, M. J. (1993). *Together we can: A guide for crafting a profamily system of education and human services.* Washington, DC: U.S. Department of Education and U.S. Department of Health and Human Services.

Mercy, J. A. (1993). Public health policy for preventing violence. *Health Affairs, 12,* 7–29.

Mihalic, S. F., Fagan, A., Irwin, K., Ballard, D., & Elliott, D. (2004). *Blueprints model program.* Boulder, CO: University of Colorado at Boulder, Center for the Study and Prevention of Violence.

National Scientific Council on the Developing Child. (2006). *Working Paper No. 3. Excessive stress disrupts the architecture of the developing brain.* Cambridge, MA: Author. Retrieved February 8, 2007, http://www.developingchild.net/pubs/wp/ Stress Disrupts Architecture Developing Brain.pdf.

Pinheiro, P. S. (2006). *World report on violence against children.* Geneva, Switzerland: United Nations.

Schechter, S., & Edleson, J. (1999). *Effective intervention in domestic violence & child maltreatment cases: Guidelines for policy and practice.* Retrieved February 8, 2007, from University of Minnesota, Violence Against Women Online Resources website: http://www.vaw.umn.edu/documents/executvi/executvi.html.

Schmidt, J. (2005). Strategic approaches to improving the well-being of children in foster care. *Voices for America's children, February.* Retrieved February 8, 2007, http:// voicesforamericaschildren.org/Content/ContentGroups/Publications-Voices/Child_Welfare2/ Strategic Approaches to Improving_the_Well-Being_of_Children_in_Foster_Care/ StrategicApproaches.pdf.

Schonkoff, J. P., & Phillips, D. A. (2000). *From neurons to neighborhoods: The science of early childhood development.* Washington, DC: National Academy Press.

Soler, M. (1992). Interagency services in juvenile justice systems. In I. Schartz (Ed.), *Juvenile justice and public policy* (pp. 134–180). New York: Lexington Books.

Straus, M. A. (1991, September). *Children as witness to maternal violence: A risk factor for life-long problems among a nationally representative sample of American men and women.* Paper presented at the Ross Round Table Children and Violence, Washington, DC.

Taylor, N., Gilbert, A., Mann, G., & Ryan, B. E. (2005). *Assessment-based treatment for traumatized children: A trauma assessment pathway.* San Diego, CA: Chadwick Center for Children & Families. Retrieved February 8, 2007, http://www.chadwickcenter. org/ Assessment-Based%20Treatment.htm

Toth, S. L., Maughan, A., Manly, J. T., Spagnola, M., & Cichetti, D. (2002). The relative efficacy of two interventions in altering maltreated preschool children's representational models: Implications for attachment theory. *Development and Psychopathology, 14*(4), 877–908.

University of Missouri-St. Louis, Children's Advocacy Services of Greater St. Louis. (2006, October). *Shifting school paradigms: Changing teacher perceptions and interventions with traumatized children.* Annual Symposium on Child Trauma, St. Louis, MO.

University of Virginia, Richmond. (2002, July). *Evaluation: Implications for cost-effective treatment for a juvenile justice population.* Retrieved February 8, 2007 from the Institute for Family Centered Services website: http://www.ifcsinc.com/brochures.

U.S. Department of Education. (1997). *Remarks by the President and the First Lady at White House Conference on Early Child Development and Learning.* Retrieved February 8, 2007, http://www.ed.gov/PressReleases/04–1997/970417d.html

U.S. Department of Justice. (2000). *Safe from the start: Taking action on children exposed to violence.* Washington, DC: Author.

Utah State University, Early Intervention Research Institute. (2005, May). *An outcomes-based approach to evaluating service coordination models.* Retrieved February 8,

2007 from the National Early Childhood TA Center website: http://nectac.org/~pdfs/topics/scoord/FINALOUTCOMESREPORT_Roberts.pdf.

Willmon-Haque, S., & Bigfoot, D. S. (2008). Violence and the effects of trauma on American Indian and Alaska Native populations. *Journal of Emotional Abuse, 8*(1/2), 51–66.

Zero to Three. (2000). *Protecting young children in violent environments: A framework to build on.* Retrieved February 8, 2007 http://www.zerotothree.org/Vol20–5.pdf

Safe Start: Promising Practices from the Evaluation of the Demonstration Project Association for the Study and Development of Community

Mary M. Hyde
Yvette H. Lamb
David Chavis

Building and disseminating knowledge about policy and practice innovations for addressing the needs of children exposed to violence represents central goals of the Safe Start Initiative (see Kracke & Cohen, 2008, this issue). Several important practice advances were made through the Safe Start Demonstration Project (Phase I of the initiative). Because children exposed to violence cross multiple service paths in their communities,

Safe Start provides resources that help local practitioners work together to respond most effectively to the problem of childhood exposure to violence. Safe Start Phase I evaluation findings illustrate the initiative's role in creating more comprehensive and responsive local service delivery systems for children exposed to violence and their families. The practices implemented as part of larger systems change strategies contributed to the knowledge-building efforts underway in the field of children exposed to violence. Safe Start Phase II (Safe Start Promising Approaches) is being evaluated through a rigorous quasi-experimental design and holds great promise for increasing the field's understanding of the most effective practice interventions for children exposed to violence in a variety of settings.

Childhood exposure to violence is a developing field with roots in both research and practice. Researchers and practitioners from diverse disciplines have focused on defining and measuring violence exposure, designs and methodologies to capture the range of children's experiences, theory, and model development for understanding potential outcomes and impact of exposure, interventions and services research, and effective policies and practices (Feerick & Silverman, 2006; Hulbert, 2008, this issue; Saunders, 2003). With the exception of Edleson's (2006) proposed system of care for children exposed to domestic violence,[1] less attention has been given to how practitioners and researchers can work together to create more responsive systems for children exposed to violence.

Practitioners and researchers had the opportunity to build such systems of care as part of the Safe Start Demonstration Project. Together they developed strategies for developing and implementing a continuum of care for children exposed to family and community violence. Over the course of Phase I of the initiative, promising practices that supported effective implementation of these strategies emerged among project participants. These promising practices are important to share with the field because they further understanding of how to effectively support a system of care for children exposed to violence.

This article highlights the promising practices developed by Safe Start Demonstration Project grantees and their partners to more effectively respond to children exposed to violence. A brief description of the Safe Start Demonstration Project is followed by an overview of the national evaluation methodology, including the specific methods used to identify promising practices. Specific practices implemented by Safe Start Demonstration Project grantees in the areas of identification, screening, referral, and interventions are described next. The article concludes with a consideration of the practices and research implications of these evaluation findings. Recommendations for future directions for the field of children exposed to violence are also presented.

THE SAFE START DEMONSTRATION PROJECT: OVERVIEW OF THE PROJECT

In 1999, the Office of Juvenile Justice and Delinquency Prevention (OJJDP) created the Safe Start Initiative. (Readers seeking a more extensive review of the Safe Start Initiative are referred to Kracke & Cohen (2008, this issue) and Hulbert (2008, this issue).) The initial phase of this comprehensive initiative was developing a demonstration project to prevent and reduce the impact of family and community violence on children 6 years and younger. The demonstration project sought to develop community-driven models of comprehensive systems that focused on improving access, delivery, and quality of services for young children who have been exposed to violence or are at high risk of exposure. Participants created strategies in the areas of service integration, enhanced programming, training, and community awareness.

METHOD

Sample

A total of 11 communities received grants from OJJDP to plan and implement a local Safe Start project: Baltimore, MD, Bridgeport, CT,

Chatham, NC, Chicago, IL, Pinellas, FL, Rochester, NY, San Francisco, CA, Spokane, WA, Washington, ME, Sitka tribe of Alaska, and the Pueblo of Zuni, NM.

Procedures

The Safe Start National Evaluation Team used several evaluation activities to discover and understand the impact of the project on children exposed to violence and their families, the systems (e.g., human services, mental health) with which they interacted, and the communities in which they lived. Promising practices were identified within the context of the initiative's national evaluation, which was guided by a theory of change (Chen, 1990; Connell & Kubisch, 1998; Connell, Kubisch, Schorr, & Weiss, 1995; Weiss, 1972). A literature review was conducted to determine criteria for selecting promising practices. It was determined that a practice was promising if as implemented it demonstrated effectiveness and success, potential for replication, and improvement over prior efforts (Association for the Study and Development of Community, 2006a). Also, promising practices had to meet criteria for standards of evidence, which included two or more independent sources (e.g., site visit discussions and reports, progress reports), high frequency of data encountered, and confirmation by Safe Start project directors. Analyses reported in three national evaluation team reports (Association for the Study and Development of Community, 2005, 2006a, 2006b) provided the foundation for the findings described below.

FINDINGS

The systems change strategies implemented by the Safe Start Demonstration Project participants were central to the multi-level theory of change guiding the initiative. These strategies were in the areas of service integration, improvement in services and interventions, training, and community awareness. It was expected that these strategies would address the challenges associated with existing service delivery systems operating in the participants' communities. The strategies were also expected to build upon the promising new directions for prevention, intervention, and treatment that were emerging in the field when the initiative started. Safe Start Demonstration Project participants implemented several promising practices that contributed to effective systems changes. Strategies and practices used to improve the identification, screening, referral, and treatment of children exposed to violence are described later. The broader systems change strategies are described first in each section and are followed by examples of promising practices from Safe Start Demonstration Project sites.

Identification, Screening, and Referral Strategies and Practices

The primary strategy for identifying, screening, and referring children exposed to violence used by the Safe Start Demonstration Project participants was the development of new screening procedures and protocols. Many child-serving agencies did not have screening procedures and protocols specifically for identifying children exposed to violence prior to the Safe Start Demonstration Project. New screening procedures ranged from instrument validation studies (e.g., testing whether or not an instrument measures what it is intended to measure), to the creation of screening forms designed specifically to detect violence exposure, to the addition of a question or code to existing forms. Using this strategy, the Safe Start Demonstration Project participants identified more than 16,000 children exposed to violence over 3 years and across 11 sites.

Five promising practices used primarily by law enforcement partners are now described. Law enforcement officers were the key point of entry into the continuum of care for all 11 Safe Start Demonstration Project participants. The practices described in Table 1 represent examples of how to make law enforcement an effective point of entry for children exposed to violence. They illustrate the importance of integrating screening practices into existing procedures in ways that minimize the documentation burden for responding officers and better prepare them for the incident once on the scene. Practice four further illustrates the need for partnering with police with the mindfulness of the first responders' needs to react quickly to a crisis and the reality of the requirement to move on to the next crisis. The last practice provides an example of how existing intake procedures can be modified to include questions about domestic violence, ensuring referrals to appropriate services.

Treatment, Service Integration, and Enhanced Programming Strategies and Practices

Safe Start Demonstration Project participants improved local community capacity for clinically treating children exposed to violence and their families by introducing evidence-based interventions into the existing

TABLE 1. Promising practices in identification, screening, and referral

Practice	Description of Practice	Safe Start Sites
Enhancing 911 for identification	In Spokane, a question was added to the 911 protocol regarding the presence of children when a domestic violence call is received. The responding police officer would receive an electronic notification. In San Francisco, a coding process for domestic violence was used in a similar fashion. In both sites, responding officers made referrals to Safe Start services.	Spokane (WA); San Francisco (CA)
Police dispatch software	In consultation with detectives of the Silver City Police Department, dispatch software was modified to document calls related to children exposed to violence, capturing the number and location of violent incidents occurring in the presence of a child 8 years or younger.	Chatham County (NC)
Digital camera project	Keeping Children Safe Downeast distributed 37 digital cameras to first responders (e.g., police officers, emergency medical personnel) to document the extent and type of injuries sustained by children to determine abuse.	Washington County (ME)
Fast response time	To increase the number of referrals from police, Spokane Safe Start implemented a practice of responding to the scene of domestic violence as fast or faster than the time it would take for a tow-truck to arrive at a collision—an average of 30 minutes, according to Spokane Safe Start research.	Spokane (WA)
Educating families and service providers for identification	Chicago Safe Start developed a partnership with the local Temporary Aide for Needy Families (TANF) to educate staff about domestic violence and screen and refer children exposed to violence. In Bridgeport, a protocol was developed and used by child protection workers to screen families for domestic violence and refer to appropriate services. The protocol was supplemented by domestic violence training for DCF staff, as well as case consultation to assist caseworkers in using the protocol and developing case plans.	Chicago (IL); Bridgeport (CT)

mental health system. While it was an effective systems change strategy, there were no identified promising practices associated with introducing evidence-based mental health treatments into communities. However, early indications are that institutionalizing this capacity by using a train-the-trainer model (Pinellas, FL; Bridgeport, CT) is an emerging promising practice.

Two primary strategies used to improve interventions and services outside of the context of therapeutic interventions are service integration and enhanced programming. Families with young children have multiple needs such as employment, housing, transportation, childcare, and individual counseling for substance and/or mental health issues. Safe Start Demonstration Project participants that provided a range of family services (rather than mental health services exclusively) engaged (i.e., identified, assessed, referred, treated) the highest number of children and families early in the initiative and were able to maintain these high numbers over time. Improving health and human services so that they engage families with multiple needs often requires service integration strategies and practices (Agranoff, 1991), such as co-locating services and sharing case information streamlined the system for families and partnering agencies. Further, developing enhanced and expanded program strategies to create a comprehensive and responsive service delivery system reduced fragmentation and centralized services access.

Four practices described in Table 2 illustrate how Safe Start participants successfully achieved service integration and engaged and retained families in services. The first practice provided coordination among service providers to reduce duplication of efforts, facilitate consideration of the whole family, and create opportunities for collective problem-solving. The other three practices exemplify the importance of engaging families in services quickly by addressing their most pressing needs as identified and prioritized by them. Making intervention and treatment convenient in both time and location helps keep families engaged in services. Finally, a central tenant of working with families experiencing violence is protecting them from further coercion, including systemic coercion that can take the form of mandating services. A high quality system of care for children exposed to violence, therefore, must be capable of providing parents the opportunity to fully participate in decisions about what services and supports are most appropriate for meeting their family's needs.

Changing service delivery systems required engagement beyond families and children exposed to violence. Raising community awareness of

TABLE 2. Promising practices in service integration
and enhanced programming

Practice	Description of Practice	Safe Start Sites
Coordinated case review	A formal review process for cross-disciplinary professional providers was developed to share information about families, conduct joint service planning, and reduce the isolation of individual service providers.	Chatham County (NC); San Francisco (CA); Washington County
Using case managers to engage families sooner	A case manager partnered with family advocates to shorten waiting times and engage families sooner. Once a family was engaged by a case manager responsible for addressing basic and immediate needs, a family advocate could start addressing therapeutic needs.	Pinellas County (FL)
Home-based therapy	Recognizing that some children exposed to violence and their families may have needs that cannot be met through family support services or clinic-based services, several sites funded intensive home-based therapy programs, in both English and Spanish. Services were provided at times that were convenient to the family, including nights and weekends.	Chatham County (NC); Bridgeport (CT); Pinellas County (FL)
Voluntary engagement during crisis	The 1st step of the "voluntary-based protocol" was for the police to get verbal permission from the family to call the Child Outreach Team (COT). The family was informed that the COT member was neither a Child Protective Service (CPS) worker nor a member of law enforcement, but a mandated reporter and must contact CPS if they think a child is in imminent danger. Voluntary engagement was viewed as critical to establishing trust and respect for engagement in a time of crisis.	Spokane (WA)

and support for children exposed to violence increased identification and linkages to appropriate services. Strategies for community action and awareness included training professionals from multiple disciplines and educating community residents.

Promising practices in the area of training and education are described in Table 3. Several Safe Start Demonstration Project participants launched successful social marketing and public education campaigns. Bridgeport and Rochester Safe Start sites obtained evidence of the campaign's influence on community response to children exposed to violence. Project participants found that addressing the issue of children exposed to violence required attention to cross-cultural issues, including racial, ethnic, gender, and organizational cultural differences that had to be bridged in order to raise awareness of children exposed to violence among all community members. The fourth practice reinforces the value of focusing training efforts on systems with the authority to influence other systems serving vulnerable families, while the last practice in Table 3 recognizes the importance of incorporating families' perspectives in training and awareness activities to ensure their relevance to those they most seek to influence.

PRACTICE IMPLICATIONS AND FUTURE DIRECTIONS

The Safe Start Demonstration Project has contributed to the field of practice for children's exposure to violence in several ways. First, the success participants experienced with law enforcement partners suggest that practitioners and policymakers may want to consider the potential for establishing a mechanism for collecting national level data regarding children's exposure to domestic violence. The practices developed by Safe Start Demonstration Project participants support the capacity of local law enforcement to make small modifications to their reporting processes that capture this data. Institutionalizing this process by creating a standard code for domestic violence and incorporating the code into the national uniform crime reporting system would benefit the field. In addition to this contribution, Safe Start Demonstration Project practices demonstrate, regardless of discipline (e.g., social services, mental health, domestic violence), the importance of working with families quickly, respectfully, and voluntarily. Providing services in this fashion insures that families with multiple needs have these needs addressed in a manner that engages and retains them in treatment and other services. Finally, the practices developed by Safe Start Demonstration Project participants show how the importance of raising public awareness using culturally competent approaches that reflect family perspectives and values has the greatest potential for changing community perspectives about violence and its impact on young children.

TABLE 3. Promising practices in community awareness and training

Practice	Description of Practice	Safe Start Sites
Public education campaigns	Social marketing and public education campaigns were developed to increase the willingness of community members to respond to children's exposure to violence.	Pinellas County (FL); Rochester (NY); San Francisco (CA); Bridgeport (CT)
Increasing cultural competence	San Francisco translated everything into Spanish and Chinese, used ethnic media and organizations to reach these communities, engaged same-gender families, initiated a dialogue with advocates and providers in the LGBT community, and encouraged members of the service delivery system to understand each other's needs and learn to speak each other's "language."	San Francisco (CA)
Incorporating tribal traditions	Zuni Safe Start focused on the use of the Zuni language and wove in Safe Start messages to bring added awareness to traditions and cultural practices.	Pueblo of Zuni (NM)
Training dependency court judges	Training judges on the issues of children exposed to violence served as a way to begin efforts to change the Department of Child and Family Services through mandated court orders (i.e., asking questions about the extent of child exposure to violence).	Spokane (WA)
Engaging parents in community awareness	A Family Engagement Study (Bridgeport) was conducted to identify barriers to services. The findings were used to develop training for staff. Parents were involved throughout the process, from designing questions to conducting analyses. In Chicago, focus groups and interviews with parents were used to develop outreach materials addressing children exposed to violence.	Bridgeport (CT); Chicago (IL)

Overall, the following opportunities are associated with the Safe Start Demonstration Project:

- The Safe Start Demonstration Project provided grantees the opportunity to put the issue of children's exposure to violence on the community's agenda and/or elevate the importance of the issue.

- The Safe Start Demonstration Project provided pilot communities with resources to enhance and integrate existing services for children and their families, and to develop those services in communities with fewer resources.
- The Safe Start Demonstration Project provided the opportunity to further legitimize the role of human service professionals as agents of change within their systems, particularly with the support of federal funding.
- Safe Start Demonstration Project grantees had the opportunity to form new working relationships, both locally and nationally.

This article represents an initial examination of the relationship between strategies and practices used to address the issue of children exposed to violence. Child exposure to violence is a developing field and there have been few systematic reviews of strategies and practices, particularly in the context of the types of systems change approaches that were undertaken by the Safe Start Demonstration Project. Therefore, more collaborative research with practitioners, policymakers, and researchers is needed in order to fully understand this relationship and improve practice.

NOTE

1. Edleson uses the term "domestic violence" solely in reference to adult-to-adult domestic violence.

REFERENCES

Agranoff, R. (1991). Human services integration: Past and present challenges in public administration. *Public Administration Review, 51*(6), 533–542.

Association for the Study and Development of Community. (2005). *Promising practices of Safe Start Demonstration Project sites: A first look.* Gaithersburg, MD: Author.

Association for the Study and Development of Community. (2006a). *Promising practices of Safe Start Demonstration Project sites: 2005.* Gaithersburg, MD: Author.

Association for the Study and Development of Community. (2006b). *Creating comprehensive and responsive systems of care for children exposed to violence: The Safe Start Demonstration Project.* Gaithersburg, MD: Author.

Chen, H. (1990). *Theory driven evaluations.* Thousand Oaks, CA: Sage Publications.

Connell, J. P., & Kubisch, A. C. (1998). Applying a theory of change approach to the evaluation of comprehensive community initiatives: Progress, prospects, and problems. In K. F. Anderson, A. C. Kubisch, & J. P. Connell (Eds.), *New approaches to evaluating community initiatives. Volume 2: Theory, measurement and analysis* (pp. 15–44). Washington, DC: The Aspen Institute.

Connell, J. P., Kubisch, A. C., Schorr L. B., & Weiss C. H. (Eds.) (1995). *New approaches to evaluating community initiatives: Concepts, methods, and contexts.* Washington, DC: The Aspen Institute.

Edleson, J. L. (2006). A response system for children exposed to domestic violence: Public policy in support of best practices. In M. Feerick & G. B. Silverman (Eds.), *Children exposed to violence* (pp. 191–211). Baltimore, MD: Brookes Publishing Company.

Feerick, M., & Silverman, G. B. (2006). *Children exposed to violence.* Baltimore, MD: Paul H. Brookes Publishing Company.

Hulbert, S. N. (2008) Children exposed to violence in the child protection system: Practice-based assessment of the system process can lead to practical strategies for improvement. *Journal of Emotional Abuse, 8*(1/2), 217–234.

Kracke, K., & Cohen, E. (2008). The Safe Start Initiative: Building and disseminating knowledge to support children exposed to violence. *Journal of Emotional Abuse, 8*(1/2), 155–174.

Saunders, B. E. (2003). Understanding children exposed to violence: Toward an integration of overlapping fields. *Journal of Interpersonal Violence, 18*(4), 356–376.

Weiss, C. H. (1972). *Evaluation research: Methods of assessing program effectiveness.* Englewood Cliffs, NJ: Prentice Hall.

Community-Based Treatment Outcomes for Parents and Children Exposed to Domestic Violence

Kimberly D. Becker
Gloria Mathis
Charles W. Mueller
Kata Issari
Su Shen Atta

Each year, approximately 10–15 million children are exposed to some form of domestic violence (McDonald, Jouriles, Ramisetty-Mikler, Caetano, & Green, 2006a; Straus, 1992). Such experiences result in clinical levels of adjustment difficulties for approximately 25–70% of children (McDonald & Jouriles, 1991). Over time, a childhood history of family violence heightens the risk for impairments in emotional and behavioral functioning (e.g., Jouriles, Spiller, Stephens, McDonald, & Swank, 2000).

The severity of problems observed in children exposed to family violence points to the need for effective treatment programs (see Gewirtz & Medhanie, 2008, this issue). It has been estimated that over 800 shelters for battered women provide programs to help children exposed to violence (Rossman, Hughes, & Rosenberg, 2000). Programs are also appearing in other arenas, including mental health and community service agencies, family courts, and hospitals (Sullivan & Allen, 2001). The most common interventions target emotional, cognitive, and behavioral difficulties experienced by these children, and many programs also provide direct services to mothers (e.g., Graham-Bermann, 1992; Jouriles et al., 2001; Sullivan, Bybee, & Allen, 2002).

Despite the importance and pervasiveness of intervention services for children experiencing domestic violence, only about a dozen outcome studies of treatment for these children have been published (outcome studies are indicated with an asterisk* in the references section), with most of them demonstrating improvement following intervention.

Graham-Bermann (2000) described three types of intervention programs: "universal" prevention, "selective" prevention (for children exposed to violence but not necessarily demonstrating problems), and "indicated" prevention (exposed to violence and manifesting difficulties, such as child behavior problems). Most clinic-based programs fall into the "selective" category (Graham-Bermann, 2000). These programs encounter a challenge in that some children exposed to family violence manifest behavioral or emotional problems while others do not. Although selective intervention programs appropriately focus on domestic violence safety or attitudinal issues, it remains unclear how many children who are at risk for long-term behavioral or emotional difficulties benefit from these sorts of programs.

At the time of Graham-Bermann's (2000) review, only one program was categorized as an "indicated" intervention (i.e., Jouriles et al., 2001). Jouriles and colleagues provided child management skills training to 36 mothers of children ages 4 to 9 exposed to domestic violence who had also been diagnosed with conduct disorder. In terms of the direct target of intervention, greater and faster improvement in child management skills was exhibited by mothers who received treatment compared to those in the control group. Additionally, though an indirect treatment target, externalizing symptoms improved for children in both groups, with children who received the intervention improving at a faster rate. Children's internalizing symptoms, which were neither a direct nor an indirect intervention target, also improved comparably whether treatment was provided or not. At a 2-year follow-up, although mean scores of externalizing and internalizing difficulties were similar across groups, significantly fewer children receiving the intervention exhibited clinically significant problems (McDonald, Jouriles, & Skopp, 2006b).

The importance of involving parents in treatment was illustrated by another study in which children who participated in a combined child and parent treatment group showed the greatest improvement, especially for externalizing symptoms, compared to children in child-only and no-treatment groups (Graham-Bermann, Lynch, Banyard, DeVoe, & Halabu, 2007). In this study of 181 children ages 6 to 12 and their mothers exposed to interpersonal violence during the previous year, children were randomly assigned to one of three community-based intervention conditions: child-only, child + mother, or wait-list control. Following a 10-week intervention program, children in the child + mother group exhibited significantly greater improvement in externalizing behavior and attitudes about violence than did children in the other two groups.

SUMMARY

The literature on treatment outcomes for children who witness family violence, while promising, remains small and incomplete. There is a need to study community-based interventions, which differ from treatments provided both in clinics and in shelters. Whereas community-based interventions provide less methodological rigor than clinic-based programs, they can provide evidence for an intervention's effectiveness, thereby promoting the generalizability of the findings. Additionally, whereas shelter services are often crisis-oriented, focusing on assisting residents with their transition back into the community, community-based programs are likely to provide counseling on domestic violence-related and emotional issues (Saathoff & Stoffel, 1999).

In addition to modality, there are other methodological considerations when evaluating intervention programs. Some studies rely on single, rather than multiple, reporters of outcomes (Graham-Bermann & Hughes, 2003). Additionally, the impact of treatment on broad-based psychopathology symptoms (that might predict long-term functioning), in addition to family violence-related issues, has been examined in only a handful of studies. In these studies, there is evidence that internalizing and externalizing problems in children might vary in their nature and degree of resolution. Even in light of statistically significant improvement, the clinical significance of treatment outcomes has not been thoroughly explored.

Finally, outcome studies have been restricted to almost exclusively Caucasian and African-American samples, so the effectiveness of interventions with individuals from other cultures and with differing views of family relationships is unknown (see Willmon-Haque & Bigfoot (2008, this issue) for an introduction to cultural issues within the American Indian population). Our own review found no published studies on treatment outcomes among predominantly Asian and Pacific Island Americans, and certainly none that attempted to incorporate Asian and Pacific Island cultural components into its program.

STUDY DESIGN AND AIMS

The present study examined child and nonoffending parental (or guardian) outcomes following participation in an established 12-week, community-based, culturally influenced intervention program involving a sample largely identifying as from Asian and Pacific Island descent. Counselor ratings of children and parents on domestic violence-related issues and parents' reports of their own parenting skills and their children's internalizing and externalizing difficulties were assessed before and immediately after completion of the program.

METHOD

Participants

Between 2001 and 2003, children from 106 families were referred to the "Haupoa Family Component," a unit of a domestic violence program within Parents And Children Together (PACT). These children were referred by their parents, or through court services, shelters for battered women, and various other programs in the community. Recruitment for the present study included random selection of one child from each family, yielding a sample size of 106 children (37 boys, 69 girls) between the ages of 3 and 17 ($M = 8.64$, $SD = 3.72$). Self-reports of ethnicity from parent participants indicated a sample of diverse ethnic backgrounds. Specifically, 52.8% identified as multi-ethnic, with most of the participants reporting blends of Caucasian, Chinese, Hawaiian, Japanese, and Filipino backgrounds. Most parents reporting a sole ethnicity (30.2%) identified as either Hawaiian (11.3% of total sample) or Caucasian (10.4%). Ethnicity data were unavailable for 17% of the participants. Of the 106 participating parents, 104 were mothers (98.1%). The majority of families participating in the program had an annual income of less than $13,000.

Although information regarding the nature of family conflict was not systematically collected at that time, 56 mothers of the 106 parents completed a 28-item conflict questionnaire based on the Conflict Tactics Scale (Straus, 1979) prior to enrolling in the intervention. The majority (75%) of mothers who completed the questionnaire reported being screamed or yelled at by her partner "frequently" or "very frequently." More than half (54.6%) of the mothers reported being punched at least once, and 35.2% indicated that they had been beaten so badly they needed to seek medical treatment. Forty percent reported being threatened with a weapon on at least one occasion, and 16.3% reported frequent or very frequent threats with a weapon. Taken together, this information suggests that families who were referred to Haupoa experienced severe and frequent levels of violence comparable to those of families involved in other studies (e.g., Graham-Bermann et al., 2007).

Program Description

The Haupoa Family Component is a community-based group intervention program for adults and children exposed to domestic violence ("haupoa" is Hawaiian for "make the ground soft for planting"). The Haupoa Family Component is housed in the Parents And Children Together (PACT) Family Peace Center, a domestic violence program providing an array of services for survivors of domestic violence as well as batterers. All children in Haupoa must have a parent, guardian, or caretaker attending one of the parent groups.

The focus of this study was the 90-minute weekly support and psycho-education group provided through Haupoa over the course of 12 weeks for children who had been exposed to domestic violence. The Haupoa children's groups were designed to provide a safe setting in which children could learn more about family violence, explore their beliefs and attitudes regarding violence, and develop or enhance healthy coping skills. Haupoa children's groups were split into five groups based on age and, for teens, gender (3–5, 6–9, 10–12 years old, and two teen groups, one for males and one for females). The curriculum, which incorporated intervention components similar to those proposed by Peled and Edleson (1992), was parallel for all groups but varied on age-appropriate topics and methods of instruction. Topics included: safety skills, trust-building, self-awareness, understanding and expressing feelings, communication, "naming" domestic violence, empathy, nonviolent conflict resolution, self-esteem, self-blame, and gender stereotypes. Group facilitators utilized many teaching techniques that reflect the cultural preference for learning through experiential activities (e.g., games, role-plays, topic-appropriate stories) and the cultural emphasis on symbolic representation (e.g., visual demonstrations using an erupting volcano to symbolize anger). Learning was reinforced by weekly review and inclusion of previous material when teaching new skills.

Parent intervention was provided weekly through a simultaneous parenting support and education group in which parents learned what their children were learning in the children's group and addressed a related topic specific to parenting the child in the aftermath of domestic violence. The purpose of the parenting group was to assist parents in helping their children cope with their exposure to domestic violence and to increase their parenting skills through information sharing and skill-building. In addition to these topics, the parenting curriculum addressed topics more relevant to the parents' own adjustment, self-esteem, and mental well-being. Most of the parents in the parenting group had previously attended a group program for survivors of domestic violence run by the same organization.

Counselors

Child and parent groups were conducted by counselors with a minimum of a high school degree and 1 year experience, although many of the counselors earned college degrees and had extensive experience working with families. Counselors also participated in 40 hours of training through the Family Peace Center.

Measures of Child Functioning

Domestic Violence-Related Skills

An 11-item counselor rating checklist of domestic violence-related skills was completed at pre- and post-intervention for each child, although not necessarily by the same counselor at each assessment point. Using a six-point scale ranging from 0 (*not at all*) to 5 (*very high*), counselors rated children on their age-appropriate skills in the following domains: (a) seems motivated to participate in program, (b) has personal support system, (c) is aware of community support networks, (d) is able to identify the impact of the abuse on self, (e) demonstrates knowledge of domestic violence and power/control dynamics, (f) is able to identify her/his own strengths, (g) participates and cooperates in activities, (h) demonstrates appropriate nonabusive behaviors, (i) able to differentiate between appropriate and inappropriate expressions of anger, (j) displays coping skills, and (k) displays congruency between behavior and affect. Five additional items were completed at post-intervention: (l) follows group guidelines and limits set by facilitators, (m) lively, attentive, and alert during group, (n) shares thoughts and feelings related to group activities, (o) is able to identify a safe person to call in dangerous situations, and (p) is able to identify a safe place to go in dangerous situations. To provide comparability across the 11-item and 16-item forms, a mean rating was calculated by summing the ratings of every item and dividing by the number of items on the form. Counselor ratings showed high reliability at pre-intervention ($\alpha = .93$) and post-intervention ($\alpha = .95$).

Child Behavior Checklist

Parents completed the Child Behavior Checklist (CBCL; Achenbach, 1991) at pre-intervention and post-intervention. For the purpose of the present study, T-scores representing CBCL internalizing and externalizing scale scores were used.

Measures of Parent Functioning

Domestic Violence-Related Skills

Counselors completed a 12-item counselor rating checklist for each parent at pre- and post-intervention. Using a six-point rating scale ranging from 0 (*not at all*) to 5 (*very high*), counselors indicated the extent to which each parent (a) demonstrates an awareness of the value of self-care, (b) has parent support system, (c) is able to identify safety needs of children, (d) is able to identify the impact of the abuse on children, (e) demonstrates knowledge of domestic violence and power/control dynamics, (f) is able to identify her/his own style and strengths as a parent, (g) demonstrates constructive, basic, communication skills as a parent, (h) demonstrates appropriate nonabusive behaviors, (i) demonstrates awareness of nonviolent discipline, (j) demonstrates understanding of positive parenting skills, (k) demonstrates awareness of family structure, appropriate rules, and consequences, and (l) recognizes that children have differing needs. The mean item rating was calculated to provide comparability with the ratings on the children's measure. Internal consistency for counselor ratings of parents were high at pre-test ($\alpha = .91$) and post-test ($\alpha = .94$).

Parenting Practices

A 25-item instrument was created by program staff to assess parenting behaviors addressed in the treatment program. These items generally reflect emotionally supportive parenting behaviors (e.g., "I discipline in a positive, firm, and consistent way" and "I listen without interrupting when my children are talking."). Parents responded to these items using a four-point scale ranging from 1 (*strongly disagree*) to 4 (*strongly agree*). For the purpose of these analyses, total scores were computed, with a possible total of 100 (see Appendix A for complete instrument). This measure showed adequate reliability at both pre-test ($\alpha = .88$) and post-test ($\alpha = .86$).

Post-intervention measures were administered primarily during the final treatment session (session 12). On occasion, families who were unable to attend session 12 completed post-treatment measures at session 11 or a week or two after session 12 when contacted by program staff.

RESULTS

Attrition

Of the 106 children enrolled in the Haupoa program, 30.1% ($n = 32$) attended all 12 sessions of the intervention. The mean number of sessions attended by participants was 8.8 ($SD = 4.17$). For the purposes of this study, youth were considered to have completed the intervention if they had attended four or more treatment sessions and had at least one measure completed at post-intervention. These criteria permitted for inclusion in the study families who had attended any four sessions, including session 12 when post-intervention measures were completed, thereby decreasing the likelihood that these families include early treatment drop-outs. Based on this criterion, 83 youth (78.3%) completed the intervention and data collection procedures, whereas 23 youth (21.7%) did not. Attendance data were not available for 17 children (16%). Nine cases with missing attendance data but with at least one post-intervention measure were included as treatment completers. On average, treatment completers attended 10.71 sessions ($SD = 2.74$).[1]

The scores of completers and noncompleters did not differ on any of the pre-intervention measures. Unfortunately, because the CBCL and parenting practices questionnaire were collected from only two noncompleters, comparison of their post-test scores in these domains could not be conducted with those children who completed the program. Counselor ratings, however, suggest that noncompleters fared worse than children who remained in treatment. Counselors rated child completers as more improved on domestic violence-related skills than child noncompleters, $t (86) = 3.54$, $p = .001$. Similarly, parents of completers were rated by counselors as more improved than were parents of noncompleters, $t (82) = 2.76, p = .007$.

Age and Gender Effects

T-tests were conducted to examine gender differences and correlations were employed to examine age effects on pre- and post-intervention CBCL scores and counselor ratings. Neither gender nor age was related to any of the pre- and post-intervention scores and ratings.

Child Outcomes

Domestic Violence-Related Skills

Paired t-tests of counselors' ratings for those youth completing the intervention ($n = 83$) indicated a significant improvement in mean item ratings of violence-related skills from pre-intervention to post-intervention, t (72) = 11.10, $p < .001$.

CBCL Internalizing and Externalizing Scales

Paired t-tests indicated a significant decrease in CBCL internalizing scores from pre-intervention to post-intervention, t (44) = 4.43, $p < .001$. Similarly, CBCL externalizing scores decreased following the intervention, t (44) = 4.80, $p < .001$. It follows then, that CBCL total scores also decreased after treatment, t (44) = 5.20, $p < .001$ (see Table 1 for pre- and post-intervention means and standard deviations). Additionally, pre/post-difference scores on the internalizing and externalizing scales of the CBCL were significantly correlated with each other, r (44) = .71, $p < .001$, and with total scale difference scores (.88 and .90, respectively).

CBCL Clinical Severity of Difficulties

As an indicator of the clinical significance of the intervention, we examined the proportion of youth whose clinically severe difficulties (T ≥ 60; Achenbach, 1991) before intervention had been reduced to nonclinical levels following the intervention. Due to missing post-intervention data,

TABLE 1. Means and standard deviations of outcome variables at pre- and post-intervention for treatment completers ($n = 83$)

Instrument	n	Pre-Intervention	Post-Intervention
Child			
CBCL internalizing	45	61.73 (11.24)	53.18 (11.60)***
CBCL externalizing	45	61.29 (12.24)	53.62 (11.47)***
CBCL total	45	63.84 (10.74)	54.98 (11.14)***
Counselor rating	73	1.62 (0.80)	2.87 (0.77)***
Parent			
Parenting practices	51	75.80 (13.18)	89.18 (8.86)***
Counselor ratings	71	1.88 (0.89)	3.88 (1.54)***

***$p < .001$.

only those 47 children with both pre- and post-intervention data were included in these analyses. Mothers' reports on the total scale of the CBCL indicated that prior to receiving services, 72.3% of children exhibited levels of psychopathology within the clinical range, compared to 36.2% of children following intervention, thereby indicating a significant decrease in the proportion of children with clinically significant post-treatment psychopathology, χ^2 (1, $N = 47$) = 10.18, $p = .001$.

Examination of the externalizing and internalizing scales of the CBCL yielded similar patterns. Specifically, 57.4% and 29.8% of children had clinically significant externalizing difficulties at pre- and post-intervention, respectively, χ^2 (1, $N = 47$) = 10.23, $p = .001$. More than one-half (53.2%) of children exhibited clinically significant internalizing difficulties at pre-intervention, compared to 21.3% at post-intervention, χ^2 (1, $N = 47$) = 3.67, $p = .055$.

Parent Outcomes

Domestic Violence-Related Skills

Counselor ratings for parents indicated significant improvement following the intervention, t (70) = 19.94, $p < .001$. Means and standard deviations for parent outcomes are presented in Table 1.

Parenting Practices

Following the intervention, parents reported significant improvement in their parenting skills, t (50) = 6.86, $p < .001$.

Child and Parent Outcomes

We examined the bivariate relationships of outcome data for each child and his/her parent enrolled in Haupoa using difference scores for pre-intervention and post-intervention counselor ratings, as well as questionnaire scores (CBCL for children, parenting questionnaires for parents). Parents' pre/post-intervention change scores on the parenting practices questionnaire were moderately correlated to their children's externalizing (r (34) = .47, $p = .006$) and total CBCL change scores (r (34) = .35, $p = .04$), although caution must be used in interpreting these results because they are based on a restricted sample of participants with complete pre-test and post-test data and likely are partially influenced by common method variance related to the parent being the reporter for both measures.

DISCUSSION

The present study examined parent and child outcomes from a community-based domestic violence intervention program conducted with primarily Asian and Pacific Island Americans. Using a pre/post-treatment design, findings point to statistically and clinically significant improvement over the course of treatment. Specifically, children's and parents' domestic violence-related skills, the primary treatment target, improved following the intervention. Parents also reported improvements in parenting skills after treatment, and it should be noted that although counselors provided discussion about parenting skills, they did not provide training on parenting strategies tailored to each individual's needs. Furthermore, children showed improvements in internalizing and externalizing difficulties at post-intervention, despite the lack of direct symptom-focused intervention in these domains. Relatedly, fewer children met clinical level criteria for internalizing or externalizing problems at post-treatment compared to pre-treatment.

The present results support and expand upon findings from other studies. The magnitude of change in internalizing and externalizing CBCL scores observed in the present study (mean change of 8.4 and 7.5, respectively) falls within the range of those reported in two other studies that used the CBCL to measure treatment outcomes (Graham-Bermann et al., 2007; Jouriles et al., 2001).[2] Although there is a need for further research, it may be that the magnitude of change in behavioral problems is a function of the specific focus of the interventions. It is now generally recognized that externalizing problems respond best to interventions that include support and training for caregivers (Kazdin, 2003), so reductions in these problems will likely be enhanced by treatments with such specific parenting components. The modest correlation between parenting practices and externalizing scores at post-test suggest that a stronger effect might be apparent if more formal parent training were provided in this setting. The extent to which internalizing symptoms in children remit with or without direct symptom-based treatment needs further examination. Like other studies, the present one found significant improvements in this area of child functioning.

The intervention studied here is best described as "selective" (Graham-Bermann, 2000) because it included children exposed to domestic violence who did and did not exhibit emotional or behavioral difficulties at the time of intervention. Reliance on mean behavior problems scores as outcome measures can distort results and make inferences difficult. As such, our finding that the percent of children exhibiting clinical levels of problems lowered over the course of treatment is important. However, some children with pre-treatment scores in the clinical range remained there after treatment. More research on factors that contribute to clinically significant improvement and on treatment innovations for these children and families is sorely needed.

This study is the first to examine treatment outcomes with predominantly Asian and Pacific Island Americans. Given that family is often thought to be the core mechanism for communicating and perpetuating cultural values, beliefs, and behaviors, the demonstration of meaningful positive outcomes among both parents and children is heartening. The extent to which treatment modifications to fit the cultural styles and needs of this group contributed to these outcomes cannot be determined from this study, but provides an avenue for future research.

It is also heartening to find that significant improvement can be found in community-based intervention settings, even without many of the advantages available in more structured research-clinic settings. Throughout child mental health, we are identifying efficacious treatments (Kazdin & Weisz, 2003), yet the ability to effectively import such treatments into complex community settings is difficult (Chorpita, 2003). The present findings support the argument that such interventions can and do work in these settings.

The use of multiple reporters for both parent and child outcomes adds strength to any conclusions. Both self-report of parenting practices and counselor judgments of parental knowledge, attitudes, and behavior improved over the course of treatment and these improvement scores were related ($r = .45$). Similarly, counselor ratings of children's domestic violence-related skills and parent ratings of externalizing difficulties improved together ($r = .31$). These findings support the assertion that parental and child outcomes improved over the course of treatment, independent of the effects of rater.

The overall contribution of the findings is strengthened by the fact that despite differences in assessment instruments, program curriculum, and program structure, our results converge with those from others who have found improvements in child adjustment and parenting practices following treatment.

Limitations

The present findings must be interpreted in light of methodological limitations. Due to the archival design of this study and natural differences in the priorities of program developers and researchers, at the outset of intervention, information was not consistently gathered regarding domestic violence characteristics (e.g., frequency, severity, timing, extent of current violence exposure); thus, it is not possible to examine whether such factors related to children's and parents' outcomes in this sample.

Additionally, the lack of a no-treatment control group leaves open the possibility that participants would have improved as time passed following their exposure to family conflict, regardless of the program's effectiveness. However, although data regarding the most recent violent incident were not systematically collected, anecdotal evidence provided by program staff suggests that contact with the abuser was variable. For example, in some families, the mother and child participated in Haupoa and their abuser participated in a related program by order of the court, suggesting recent family conflict. In other families, study staff was instructed not to contact mothers by phone out of fear of the abusive live-in partner. Yet in other families, abusers were incarcerated or mothers avoided contact, suggesting more distal family conflict relative to the previous scenarios. Variability with regard to contact with abuser has been widely reported and, in fact, continued contact between families and their abusers appears to be normative in treatment studies (Graham-Bermann et al., 2007; Jouriles et al., 2001; McDonald et al., 2006b). Moreover, Jouriles and colleagues (2001; McDonald et al., 2006b) found that although approximately 40% of women experienced recurrent violence either during treatment or during the follow-up period, recurrent violence was not associated with children's treatment outcomes.

An additional threat to the internal validity of the study involves attrition of study participants. The concern is that participants who fare well during the intervention remain in treatment longer than those who do not experience improvement; thus, the treatment effects reported may be stronger than they would be if treatment dropouts had remained in the study. This is a concern in the current study because the attrition rate is 22%. At the same time, however, we hoped that including the relatively few participants with low attendance would build in a bit of conservatism in what is not a well-controlled study.

Although the inclusion of reports from multiple informants is a strength of this study, two associated limitations deserve mention. First, shared method variance as a result of having parents and clinicians report on multiple surveys likely contributes to the statistically significant correlations, such as those between parenting practices and child CBCL scores. Although other assessment methods such as behavior observations or teacher ratings would have been helpful, such data were not available for the present study.

Second, reporting biases on the part of the clinicians and parents, who invested time and energy into each child's treatment, may partially account for positive treatment outcomes. While reliance on parent or therapist judgments is common in the literature (e.g., Graham-Bermann et al., 2007; Jouriles et al., 2001; Sullivan et al., 2002; Wagar & Rodway, 1995), the use of independent evaluators blind to assessment timing, would have strengthened the study. At the same time, however, a review of the post-treatment ratings by clinicians and parents indicates opportunity for continued growth. For example, at post-treatment, the mean clinicians' rating for children was 2.87 on a scale for which 5.00 indicates mastery of treatment-related domains, and clinicians' ratings for parents also indicated room for improvement. Additionally, CBCL scores indicated approximately one-quarter of children continued to exhibit clinically significant externalizing or internalizing difficulties at post-treatment.

CONCLUSION

Given the long-term implications of domestic violence for both children's adjustment and parenting, these results suggest that children and parents can exhibit improvement in these domains following their involvement in a time-limited, community-based intervention (see Chamberlain (2008, this issue) for a discussion on community-based efforts). Moreover, it appears that improvement in functioning in these areas can ensue even with limited clinical attention specifically paid to particular symptoms or parenting challenges.

Avenues for future research are numerous in the area of domestic violence interventions. As the field accumulates evidence for the effectiveness of treatment programs, identification of the mechanisms of change will assist the field in developing evidence-based practices for children and parents exposed to intimate partner violence (IPV). Related distillation research would help illuminate the core components of treatment that bring about change in children's functioning. For example, research suggests that domestic violence treatments with parent components are more effective than those without (e.g., Graham-Bermann et al., 2007). Researchers should also endeavor to systematically examine potential cultural differences in perceptions of violence, parenting practices, and family structures that may be related to children's adjustment and that may need to be addressed in treatment programs. Finally, longitudinal studies looking at long-term adjustment following intervention are necessary to determine whether treatment gains can be maintained past childhood as youth exposed to IPV enter adolescence and adulthood.

NOTES

1. Analyses based on other criteria, such as minimum 8-session attendance for classification as "completer" and exclusion of the eight youth with post-treatment parent data but missing attendance data, did not substantively affect the results. Data analyses are available from the authors upon request.

2. Jouriles et al. (2001) reported mean change scores on the CBCL of 10.2 and 9.3 for internalizing and externalizing difficulties, respectively. Although these change scores are slightly greater in magnitude found in the current study, it should be noted that the time period between pretest and posttest was 8 months, more than twice as long as in the current study. If the change scores from the second assessment (4 months) in Jouriles et al. (2001) are used as a comparison, the magnitude of change is quite similar to that found in the current study (mean change of 9.2 and 7.6, respectively).

3. Asterisks (*) indicate family violence treatment outcome study.

REFERENCES[3]

Achenbach, T. M. (1991). *Manual for the child behavior checklist/4–18 and 1991 profile.* Burlington, VT: University of Vermont, Department of Psychiatry.

Chamberlain, L. (2008). Ten lessons learned in Alaska: Home visitation and intimate partner violence. *Journal of Emotional Abuse, 8*(1/2), 205–216.

Chorpita, B. F. (2003). The frontier of evidence-based practice. In A. Kazdin & J. Weisz (Eds.), *Evidence-based psychotherapies for children and adolescents* (pp. 42–59). New York: Guilford.

Gewirtz, A. H., & Medhanie, A. (2008). Proximity and risk in children's witnessing of domestic violence incidents. *Journal of Emotional Abuse, 8*(1/2), 67–82.

Graham-Bermann, S. A. (1992). *The Kids' Club: A preventive intervention program for children of battered women.* Ann Arbor, MI: University of Michigan, Department of Psychology.

*Graham-Bermann, S. A. (2000). Evaluating interventions for children exposed to family violence. *Journal of Aggression, Maltreatment, and Trauma, 4*, 191–215.

Graham-Bermann, S. A., & Hughes, H. M. (2003). Intervention for children exposed to interpersonal violence (IPV): Assessment of needs and research priorities. *Clinical Child and Family Psychology Review, 6*, 189–204.

*Graham-Bermann, S. A., Lynch, S., Banyard, V., DeVoe, E. R., & Halabu, H. (2007). Community-based intervention for children exposed to intimate partner violence: An efficacy trial. *Journal of Consulting and Clinical Psychology, 75*, 199–209.

*Jouriles, E. N., McDonald, R., Spiller, L., Norwood, W., Swank, P., Stephens, N., et al. (2001). Reducing conduct problems among children of battered women. *Journal of Consulting and Clinical Psychology, 69*, 774–785.

Jouriles, E. N., Spiller, L., Stephens, N., McDonald, R., & Swank, P. (2000). Variability in adjustment of children of battered women: The role of child appraisals of interparent conflict. *Cognitive Therapy and Research, 24*, 233–249.

Kazdin, A. (2003). Problem-solving skills training and parent management training for conduct disorder. In A. Kazdin & J. Weisz (Eds.), *Evidence-based psychotherapies for children and adolescents* (pp. 241–262). New York: Guilford.

Kazdin, A., & Weisz, J. (2003). *Evidence-based psychotherapies for children and adolescents.* New York: Guilford.

McDonald, R., & Jouriles, E. N. (1991). Marital aggression and child behavior problems: Research findings, mechanisms, and intervention strategies. *The Behavior Therapist, 14*, 189–192.

*McDonald, R., Jouriles, E. N., Ramisetty-Mikler, S., Caetano, R., & Green, C. E. (2006a). Estimating the number of American children living in partner-violence families. *Journal of Family Psychology, 20*, 137–142.

*McDonald, R., Jouriles, E. N., & Skopp, N. (2006b). Reducing conduct problems among children brought to battered women's shelters: Intervention effects 24 months following termination of services. *Journal of Family Psychology, 20*, 127–136.

*Peled, E., & Edleson, J. L. (1992). Multiple perspectives on groupwork with children of battered women. *Violence and Victims, 7*, 327–346.

Rossman, B., Hughes, H., & Rosenberg, M. (2000). Treatment and prevention of the impact of exposure. In B. Rossman, H. Hughes, & M. Rosenberg (Eds.), *Children and interparental violence: The impact of exposure* (pp. 107–138). Philadelphia: Taylor & Francis.

Saathoff, A., & Stoffel, E. (1999). Community-based domestic violence services [Special issue: Domestic violence and children]. *Future of Children, 9*, 97–110.

Straus, M. A. (1979). Measuring intrafamily conflict and violence: The Conflict Tactics (CT) Scales. *Journal of Marriage & the Family, 41*, 75–88.

Straus, M. A. (1992). Children as witnesses to marital violence: A risk factor for lifelong problems among a nationally representative sample of American men and women. *Report of the Twenty-Third Ross Roundtable.* Columbus, OH: Ross Laboratories.

Sullivan, C. M., & Allen, N. E. (2001). Evaluating coordinated community responses for abused women and their children. In S. A. Graham-Bermann & J. L. Edleson (Eds.), *Domestic violence in the lives of children: The future of research, intervention, and social policy* (pp. 422–447). Washington, DC: APA Books.

*Sullivan, C., Bybee, D., & Allen, N. (2002). Findings from a community-based program for battered women and their children. *Journal of Interpersonal Violence, 17*, 915–936.

*Wagar, J. M., & Rodway, M. R. (1995). An evaluation of a group treatment approach for children who have witnessed wife abuse. *Journal of Family Violence, 10*, 295–306.

Willmon-Haque, S., & Bigfoot, D. S. (2008). Violence and the effects of trauma on American Indian and Alaska Native populations. *Journal of Emotional Abuse, 8*(1/2), 51–66.

APPENDIX A

Parenting Practices Instrument

1. I take time to meet my physical and emotional needs.
2. I take time to have fun with each of my children.
3. I praise each of them for their own uniqueness.
4. My children are clear about the rules and structure in our home.
5. I am aware of age-appropriate and logical consequences.
6. I discipline in a positive, firm, and consistent way.
7. I avoid making threats and intimidating my children.
8. Each of my children has age-appropriate responsibilities.
9. I show my children that it's okay for them to make mistakes.
10. I don't compare my children to others.
11. I model appropriate ways to express anger and resolve conflict.
12. I discipline by using methods other than physical punishment.
13. I believe children who witness abuse between their parents suffer emotionally.
14. I believe children who are surrounded by parental abuse are traumatized by it.
15. I tell them that they are not responsible for any abuse (past or present).
16. I believe that using physical punishment gives them the message that violence is acceptable.
17. I do not give in to my children's inappropriate demands regardless of their behavior.
18. I allow my children to make appropriate decisions as long as safety is not an issue.
19. I acknowledge and validate my children's feelings and actions.
20. I listen without interrupting when my children are talking.
21. I know where to go for support and information regarding parenting.
22. Our family has weekly "family time."
23. I help my children understand the importance of helping others.
24. Our family observes spiritual and/or cultural traditions.
25. I am familiar with the laws and consequences regarding children's and parents' rights.

Ten Lessons Learned in Alaska: Home Visitation and Intimate Partner Violence

Linda Chamberlain

Home visitation has become an increasingly popular, community-based strategy to prevent child maltreatment and promote healthy child development and healthy family environments. There is growing interest in how the home visitation model can be adapted to help parents that are being victimized by an intimate partner and children exposed to intimate partner violence (IPV). Home visitation models vary significantly in terms of goals, philosophical orientation, the type of service providers involved, eligibility requirements, how clients are enrolled, and the range and intensity of services offered. These models typically employ nurses and/or paraprofessionals as home visitors. Participation is voluntary and at-risk families are usually recruited around the time of pregnancy or delivery. Home visitors provide a wide array of services, including assessments, education, support, and linkage to community resources. Home visitation services are often provided for several years after the birth of the target child.

A common theme that has emerged among home visitation programs is the need to systematically address IPV. One-third or more of home-visited families disclosed current or past victimization by an intimate partner (Duggan et al., 2004; El-Kamary et al., 2004; Fergusson, Hildegard, Horwood, & Ridder, 2005; Olds, Kitzman, et al., 2004b). Intimate partner violence is highly correlated with key risk factors that are used to identify families in need of home visitation services, particularly perinatal complications and child maltreatment (Berenson, Wiemann, Wilkinson, Jones, & Anderson, 1994; Rumm, Cummings, Krauss, Bell, & Rivara, 2000; Shumway et al., 1999). Intimate partner violence has been shown to reduce the effectiveness of home visitation services in preventing child abuse and neglect: over a 15-year period, the reduction in the number of reports to child protection services decreased as the frequency of IPV increased among home-visited clients who disclosed IPV compared to nurse-visited clients without IPV (Eckenrode et al., 2000). The limiting effect of IPV on the effectiveness of home visitation was not restricted to the more severe physical forms of IPV in this study population.

A few studies have examined how IPV is addressed within the context of home visitation. Duggan et al. (2004) reported that there was no documentation in clients' charts for more than 75% of home-visited families that disclosed victimization by an intimate partner (for a discussion of the invisibility of children, see Gewirtz & Medhanie (2008, this issue)). The referral rates to community services for clients who disclosed IPV remained minimal throughout the 3-year study. Tandon, Parillo, Jenkins, and Duggan (2005) conducted interviews with clients and home visitors at four different home visitation programs in Baltimore, Maryland, to examine how paraprofessional and nurse home visitors addressed IPV with pregnant and parenting women. Among home-visited women who disclosed physical or emotional abuse by a current partner, approximately one-fifth (19%) accessed IPV-related services. There was no significant difference in home visitors' communication about IPV with mothers who disclosed abuse compared to mothers who had not disclosed abuse. One-third of home visitors did not feel that they were adequately trained to address IPV with clients.

An in-depth evaluation of Healthy Families Alaska (HFAK) identified several persistent problems in addressing IPV over the 5-year study period (Alaska State Department of Health and Social Services, 2005). Modeled after a well-established, national child abuse prevention program to prevent child abuse and neglect, HFAK offered home visitation services to at-risk families that were screened for risk factors around the time of pregnancy. Families that screened positive were offered home visitation services. Families enrolled prenatally were offered at least one visit per month, while families enrolled postnatally were offered weekly visits, which could then be adjusted according to family functioning based on periodic assessments. Home visitation services were offered to families for 3 to 5 years depending on their needs.

With the exception of one program where public health nurses provided home visits, HFAK employed paraprofessionals as home visitors. The primary goals of HFAK mirrored the national program: to identify overburdened families in need of support, build trusting relationships and improve the family's support systems, teach problem-solving skills, improve the family's support system, promote positive parent-child interaction, and promote healthy child development. Healthy Families Alaska identified IPV as a malleable risk factor for child maltreatment and an outcome indicator for their programs.

While HFAK achieved many significant milestones, including that home-visited families were less likely to have extremely poor home environments for child learning, lower levels of parenting stress, greater knowledge of child development, and greater empathy toward their children, home visitation did not prevent child maltreatment or reduce malleable parent risks for maltreatment including IPV in this randomized controlled trial. Several major shortcomings in addressing IPV were identified. While nearly one-half (49%) of mothers disclosed physical IPV at the time of the baseline assessment, the majority of home visitors did not address IPV with home-visited families over the 5-year study period. Home-visited clients who experienced IPV were not any more likely to receive services for IPV than families experiencing IPV that did not received home visitation. Approximately 25% of home-visited mothers who disclosed IPV had discussed domestic violence/community referrals with their home visitor within 6 months of enrolling in the program. These findings were the catalyst for a special initiative to enhance HFAK's response to IPV.

SPECIAL INITIATIVE ON HOME VISITATION AND IPV

Healthy Families Alaska partnered with the Alaska Family Violence Prevention Project over a 2-year period to provide training and technical assistance on addressing IPV within the context of home visitation. All six of the HFAK sites that were operational from 2003–2005 participated in this initiative. Program locations ranged from larger communities (Anchorage [two program sites], Fairbanks, Juneau) to smaller and rural communities (Kenai and Palmer). Programs varied significantly in terms of the number of staff, the cultural and ethnic diversity of clients served, and the availability of IPV-related services in each locality (see Becker, Mathis, Mueller, Issari, & Atta, 2008; Gewirtz & Medhanie, 2008; and Willmon-Haque & Bigfoot, 2008, each in this issue).

The director of the Alaska Family Violence Prevention Project conducted a baseline needs assessment by telephone with each of the HFAK program directors. Health Families Alaska staff and home visitors were encouraged to participate in the needs assessment. Topics covered in the assessment included screening and intervention practices for IPV, barriers to screening and referrals, prior IPV training and training needs, and concerns about addressing IPV during home visits. The results were used to develop site-specific training and technical assistance that was responsive to each program's needs. The needs assessment process initiated an interactive dialogue with HFAK staff that promoted a reciprocal learning process.

Each program site received two site visits over the 24-month period. The first site visit focused on training staff and building partnerships. Healthy Families Alaska programs were encouraged to invite other agencies including IPV programs, public health, and child protection services to participate in the site visit and training. An advocate from an IPV agency presented information about local resources as part of each training. Meetings were held with the HFAK program director and staff at the beginning of the site visit to review the needs assessment results and adjust training based on emerging issues and concerns. Training content was adjusted to meet the needs of the local program. Due to the high turn-over of paraprofessional home visitor staff, an introductory overview of the prevalence and patterns of IPV was included in several locations. While a number of HFAK staff had prior training on early brain development, this initiative provided the first training that they had received on childhood exposure to violence and traumatic brain development. The didactic segments of the training were offered in the morning, while afternoons were dedicated to interactive discussions on screening and intervention strategies. Each program site was asked to provide a case scenario on IPV that had posed challenges for home visitors. The case scenario became the centerpiece of a problem-solving discussion to identify innovative strategies for addressing IPV during home visits. Defining success for addressing IPV within the context of home visitation was a key component of the training to help home visitors differentiate between inappropriate responses (e.g., telling a client to leave her abusive partner versus asking a client what she wanted to do about her situation), discussing safety planning, and other supportive responses.

Resource packets were sent to each of the programs following the site visit. Contents of the packet varied according to program needs but typi-cally included assessment tools, posters, safety cards, research articles, and videos. Technical assistance (TA) was provided via e-mail and tele-phone to address emerging challenges, concerns, and feedback. During the second year of the initiative, each program received a follow-up site visit that typically focused on refining assessment strategies, integrating assessment and intervention into existing practices, working on protocols for IPV, and problem-solving. Follow-up discussions on case scenarios were used to identify promising practices and new challenges. Additional resources were provided to programs on an as-needed basis. The follow-ing discussion focuses on lessons learned during this initiative to promote a systematic response to IPV within the context of home visitation.

SKILL-BASED TRAINING

Intimate partner violence was not part of the core curriculum that was used to train HFAK staff. While some home visitors had received basic IPV training, there was a persistent gap in knowledge and skills due to the high turnover among paraprofessional staff. A consistent theme that emerged during the needs assessments and dialogue with home visitors was the need to go beyond "IPV 101" to provide skill-based training on assessment and intervention. Home visitors needed to know practical strategies of how to be supportive of clients that choose not to leave a violent relationship or return to their abusive partners, how to help clients who accept violence as a norm, how to promote a positive, nonjudgmental approach to IPV with families, and how to engage fathers in prevention.

Building trusting relationships with families was central to the mission of HFAK. Home visitors stressed the importance of developing empathetic, supportive strategies to discuss this sensitive topic with families without compromising trust. Home visitors' ongoing contact with parents provided a unique opportunity to educate families about healthy relationships, while integrating information about warning signs of abusive behaviors. This approach offered a less threatening venue to discuss unhealthy relationships and abusive behaviors with clients. All of the programs offered some type of parenting skills activities which provided an opportunity to incorporate information on healthy relationships, the effects of violence on children, and information on how victimization can impact parenting. Home visitors were particularly interested in using resources from the Family Violence Prevention Fund's "Coaching Boys Into Men" campaign to engage fathers in a positive role to prevent relationship violence.

Feedback from HFAK staff indicated that defining success was a key strategy to promote empathy, prevent burnout, and help home visitors to work with clients to identify options when clients chose not to leave a violent relationship or returned to an abuser. Home visitors found that asking clients what they did to keep themselves and their children safe helped clients to identify their strengths, engage in safety planning, and recognize how the abuse affected their daily lives. Home visitors' understanding of their clients' needs facilitated an interactive process with clients to identify and implement innovative, supportive interventions. For example, one program was working with a mother and son who had significant exposure to violence. The son displayed many symptoms associated with childhood exposure to violence but the mother did not recognize the need for therapeutic intervention, did not trust therapists, and refused referrals. The home visitor worked with a local therapist to arrange a mothers' quilting event and invited the mother, an accomplished quilter, to help with the event. The mother met the therapist in a nonthreatening environment, a trusting relationship was formed, and the mother and son followed through with referrals to the therapist. Feedback indicated that when home visitors redefined success as a client feeling safer to disclose IPV and discuss options, home visitors felt more positive about their role and were able to be more supportive.

Lessons learned:

1. Home visitors need ongoing opportunities for skill-based training that addresses situations that are likely to occur in the context of home visitation.
2. Approaches such as promoting healthy relationships and positive roles for men should be part of home visitors' toolkit for addressing IPV with families.
3. Defining success for assessment and intervention for IPV within the context of home visitation should be a key component of skill-based training.

ASSESSMENT

Most of the HFAK programs did not have a written protocol that specifically addressed screening for IPV. Screening practices varied significantly from program to program in terms of the types of questions used, whether actual wording for the IPV question was provided or the home visitor was instructed to ask about "abuse," the frequency of screening, and documentation practices. Inquiry about IPV was usually limited to physical abuse. Asking clients about IPV during home visits posed some unique challenges. Spouses, partners, children, and other family members were often present during home visits. Home visitors employed a number of strategies to be able to screen the mother alone such as waiting until a follow-up visit when no one else was present or coordinating with another service provider who would be more likely to see the mother alone to conduct the screening. Some assessment strategies raised safety concerns, such as screening both parents and asking the male spouse or partner first to see how he reacts before screening the mother.

During the first year of the initiative, a compendium of IPV assessment tools developed for the clinical setting were provided to HFAK staff. A number of home visitors reported that these questions did not work with their clients. The questions were often too direct, particularly during early contact with new families when the home visitor was trying to build trust with clients that were often fearful of getting involved with government agencies. Home visitors also expressed concerns about the cultural relevancy of standardized screening questions for IPV (see Willmon-Haque

& Bigfoot, 2008, this issue). They stressed the importance of listening to the words that clients used to talk about abuse and the need to use those words when talking with clients about IPV.

Home visitors noted the need for less direct ways to talk to clients about IPV, the importance of listening carefully to clients for clues of what was going on in their lives, and strategies to ease into the topic by talking about relationships. Health Families of Alaska staff identified resources that would help them to implement routine assessment for IPV during home visits. They requested scripts that would help them to explain to clients why they were asking about relationship violence and what to say to clients when abuse was disclosed. Another common theme was the need for an assessment tool designed for home visits that offered a range of questions that could be adapted by the home visitor. Some home visitors suggested a two-tiered approach to screening, where the first tier had general questions about relationships and the second tier had questions more directly focused on IPV and unhealthy relationships.

Lessons learned:

4. IPV assessment tools that were developed for clinical settings may not be appropriate for home visits (see Gewirtz & Medhanie, 2008, this issue).
5. Home visitors need screening protocols for IPV that address circumstances and barriers associated with screening in the home setting (see Becker et al., 2008, this issue).

PROMOTING PARTNERSHIPS

Home visitors expressed frustration about the lack of resources for clients experiencing IPV and barriers to making referrals due to lack of transportation, waiting lists, and cultural considerations such as language barriers. At most of the program sites, home visitors and advocates had not met previously and often did not understand the full range of services that one another provided. Including advocates in the training and site visit activities provided a foundation to build ongoing relationships between local shelters and home visitation programs that were mutually beneficial. Home visitors described what a difference it made to be able to put a name or face to the advocate that they were referring their clients to. This personal connection helped home visitors to more successfully promote these referrals to clients. Advocates learned about home visitation services that could be offered to their clients. Strategies such as consulting with an advocate when a home visitor was unsure of how to proceed with a client experiencing IPV and inviting advocates to brown bag lunch discussions provided new venues to enhance knowledge, introduce new staff, and sustain partnerships.

Lessons learned:

6. Developing partnerships between home visitors and IPV advocates/ agencies can facilitate referrals and intervention with families experiencing IPV.
7. IPV advocates/agencies can be an ongoing resource for IPV training and case consultation.

ADDRESSING STAFF NEEDS

Home visitation poses some unique safety concerns relative to IPV. Home visitors described concerns about arriving during an IPV incident or being present as the abuse escalated. While all of the HFAK programs had general protocols for conducting home visits, these protocols did not specifically address safety concerns associated with IPV. Through brainstorming sessions, home visitors identified a variety of strategies they employed to enhance their personal safety in potentially violent households. These strategies included teaming up with another home visitor to visit the household, wearing slip-on shoes that can be put on quickly, keeping car keys and a cell phone readily accessible, checking-in with the home office upon arrival and departure, and being observant of any signs or sounds of conflict before entering the household. One program, which had invited local law enforcement to conduct safety training with their staff, learned about strategies that police use such as backing the vehicle into the driveway to allow for a quick exit. A list of safety strategies were compiled from brainstorming sessions and shared during follow-up site visits with the programs.

The high prevalence of IPV among home-visited clients, the ongoing contact and connection that home visitors have with clients, and working in the home setting where home visitors are more likely than other service providers to witness abuse and the after-effects raises major concerns about burn-out and vicarious trauma. A number of home visitors disclosed a history of victimization during site visits. Some HFAK staff described how a client's disclosure of abuse could rekindle traumatic memories. Home visitors stressed the importance of promoting self-care and boundary-setting and the need for debriefing sessions, particularly after traumatic events such as a client being seriously battered. Healthy Families of Alaska staff identified several supportive strategies, including monthly IPV case reviews, weekly debriefing sessions, and stress management training for staff.

Addressing staff's needs and safety is a key step to enhancing a program's response to IPV. While most of the programs had some type of written policy on work safety, these protocols did not address IPV in the workplace. Healthy Families of Alaska programs were advised to expand their protocols to address safety concerns associated with IPV, including stalking, threats, and harassment at work. In addition, managers were encouraged to work with employee assistance programs to ensure that trauma-informed services were available and that HFAK staff was well informed about the availability of these confidential services.

Lessons learned:

8. Home visitation protocols need to be expanded to explicitly address safety concerns associated with IPV.
9. Resources and strategies are needed to address and prevent burn-out and vicarious trauma associated with addressing IPV.
10. Workplace safety protocols should incorporate policies on IPV in the workplace.

CONCLUSION

Intimate partner violence is very prevalent among families receiving home visitation services. Home visitors have a unique opportunity to identify and address IPV through ongoing contact with families. This extraordinary window of opportunity poses significant risks and challenges unique to home visitation that should be addressed systematically with training and protocols. Safety concerns for clients and home visitors are paramount to developing protocols and policies on addressing IPV within the context of home visitation. This special initiative identified several key considerations to help inform protocol and policy development, including the need for skill-based training and IPV assessment tools that are developed and piloted in the home setting, the importance of developing partnerships between home visitors and IPV advocates/agencies, and the need to address vicarious trauma, safety issues during home visitation, and IPV as a workplace safety issue. The lessons learned through this initiative were instrumental in designing an assessment tool to help home visitation programs evaluate their progress in developing a coordinated response to IPV. The tool will be available to home visitation programs nationwide.

The wide range of services that can be offered by home visitors including assessment, parenting skills, and referrals to community-based agencies can provide new inroads to reaching victimized parents and children growing up in violent households. Home visitors frequently have contact with fathers and other males in the household, which can be an avenue to prevention. As home visitation programs enhance their response to IPV, home visits may become a promising practice to reduce and prevent IPV. In a large-scale randomized trial in Denver, Colorado, nurse-visited women reported less physical violence from partners in the past 6 months compared to controls (Olds et al., 2004a). What is especially noteworthy is that the effect of home visitation on IPV was measured 2 years after home visitation services had ended.

REFERENCES

Alaska State Department of Health and Social Services. (2005). *Evaluation of the Healthy Families Alaska Program: Final report*. Anchorage, AK: Author.

Becker, K. D., Mathis, G., Mueller, C. W., Issari, K., & Atta, S. S. (2008). Community-based treatment outcomes for parents and children exposed to domestic violence. *Journal of Emotional Abuse, 8*(1/2), 187–204.

Berenson, A. B., Wiemann, C. M., Wilkinson, G. S., Jones, W. A., & Anderson, G. D. (1994). Perinatal morbidity associated with violence experienced by pregnant women. *American Journal of Obstetrics and Gynecology, 170*, 1760–1769.

Duggan, A., Fuddy, L., Burrell, L., Higman, S. M., McFarlane, E., Windham, A., et al. (2004). Randomized trial of a statewide home visiting program to prevent child abuse: Impact in reducing parental risk factors. *Child Abuse & Neglect, 28*, 623–643.

Eckenrode, J., Ganzel, B., Henderson, C. R., Smith, E., Olds, D. L., Powers, J., et al. (2000). Preventing child abuse and neglect with a program of nurse home visitation: The limiting effects of domestic violence. *Journal of the American Medical Association, 184*(11), 1385–1391.

El-Kamary, S. S., Higman, S. M., Fuddy, L., McFarlane, E., Sia, C., & Duggan, A. K. (2004). Hawaii's Health Start Home Visiting Program: Determinants and impact of rapid repeat birth. *Pediatrics, 114*, 317–326.

Fergusson, D. M., Hildegard, G. L., Horwood, J., & Ridder, E. M. (2005). Randomized trial of the early start program of home visitation. *Pediatrics, 116*, 803–809.

Gewirtz, A. H., & Medhanie, A. (2008). Proximity and risk in children's witnessing of domestic violence incidents. *Journal of Emotional Abuse, 8*(1/2), 67–82.

Olds, D. L., Robinson, J., Pettitt, L., Luckey, D. W., Holmberg, J., Ng, R. K., et al. (2004a). Effects of home visits by paraprofessionals and by nurses: Age 4 follow-up results of a randomized trial. *Pediatrics, 114*(6), 1560–1568.

Olds, D. L., Kitzman, H., Cole, R., Robinson, J., Sidora, K., Luckey, D. W., et al. (2004b). Effects of nurse home-visiting on maternal life course and child development: Age 6 follow-up results of a randomized trial. *Pediatrics, 114*(6), 1550–1558.

Rumm, P. D., Cummings, P., Krauss, M. R., Bell, M. A., & Rivara, F. P. (2000). Identified spouse abuse as a risk factor for child abuse. *Child Abuse and Neglect, 11*, 1375–1381.

Shumway, J., O'Campo, P., Gielen, A., Witter, F. R., Khouzami, A. N., & Blakemore, K. J. (1999). Preterm labor, placental abruption, and premature rupture of membranes in relation to maternal violence or verbal abuse. *The Journal of Maternal-Fetal Medicine, 8*, 76–80.

Tandon, S. J., Parillo, K. M., Jenkins, C., & Duggan, A. K. (2005). Formative evaluation of home visitors' role in addressing poor mental health, domestic violence, and substance abuse among low-income pregnant and parenting women. *Maternal and Child Health Journal, 9*(3), 273–283.

Willmon-Haque, S., & Bigfoot, D. S. (2008). Violence and the effects of trauma on American Indian and Alaska Native populations. *Journal of Emotional Abuse, 8*(1/2), 51–66.

FUTURE DIRECTION

Children Exposed to Violence in the Child Protection System: Practice-Based Assessment of the System Process can Lead to Practical Strategies for Improvement

Serena N. Hulbert

IDENTIFYING THE NEED: CHILDREN EXPOSED TO DOMESTIC VIOLENCE AND CHILD PROTECTION

Over the past few decades, professionals have increased their awareness of the co-occurrence of domestic violence and child maltreatment and its impact.[1] Research indicates that children exposed to violence are at an increased risk of being abused or neglected. A majority of studies reveal there are adult and child victims in 30–60% of families experiencing domestic violence.[2] Many children and parents coming into contact with the child protection system are also often being subjected to domestic violence along with other co-occurring factors, creating an overlapping problem for all professionals working in the child protection system.

Increased awareness regarding the co-occurrence of domestic violence and child abuse compels child protection and domestic violence professionals to re-evaluate their services and interventions with families experiencing multiple forms of violence. Although adult and child victims are often found in the same families, child protection and domestic violence professionals have divergent responses to the child and the adult, largely due to differences in each system's development, philosophy, mandates, policies, and practices.[3]

COLLABORATIVE APPROACHES TO CHILD PROTECTION SYSTEM IMPROVEMENT

In response to emerging statistics and research on the prevalence and effects of violence on children, the Office of Juvenile Justice and Delinquency Prevention (OJJDP) of the U.S. Department of Justice worked with federal partners in the Office of Justice Programs and the U.S. Department of Health and Human Services to develop the Safe Start

Initiative (Safe Start). The purpose of the initiative is to prevent and reduce the impact of family and community violence on children.[4]

Four years ago in several Safe Start demonstration sites, discussions began regarding ways to improve how the child protection system identifies, assesses, and treats families co-experiencing domestic violence and child abuse and neglect. Professionals were looking for practical ways in which they could improve coordination among the child welfare, domestic violence, and legal/court systems. One query that was raised by stakeholders in all the jurisdictions was whether the child protection system removes children from their primary caregiver based solely or primarily on one factor: the children have witnessed domestic violence. Research funded in four diverse jurisdictions allowed for the development of a research design and tools that provided a means to practically assess how the child protection system manages cases. By evaluating the way child protection systems identify, assess, and treat families experiencing violence, stakeholders can use concrete data instead of anecdotal evidence to improve practices.

The research design needed to assess the impact that policies and procedures had on the child protection case flow in order to determine whether particular practices could be identified that were influencing the outcomes for children and families. System-wide research took place in varying degrees in Chatham County, NC; Pinellas County, FL; San Francisco, CA; and Spokane, WA. From 2002–2006, data were collected from 582 dependency court case files and departments of social services files in the four jurisdictions. Over 100 system stakeholders, domestic violence victims, and parents in the child protection system were interviewed or surveyed in the jurisdictions during more than 36 site visits.

Data collection instruments were developed by focusing on the "big picture" of the system's management of child protection cases and focused primarily on families whose situations required involvement with the dependency court. The "big picture" involved looking at the way in which entities interacted and their policies and practices overlapped. Stakeholders in the four jurisdictions wanted data that would help them focus resources and problem-solving efforts on concrete problems rather than perceived issues. Many stakeholders commented on how difficult it is to improve how the system handles cases when new or revised system policies and procedures are based on anecdotal evidence or are reactions to a crisis.

This research design was tailored specifically to each jurisdiction by identifying the statutory and policy framework in which the child protection system operates, which allowed for identification of gaps or inconsistencies in how the system manages cases rather than focusing on or assuming that outcomes were influenced only by philosophies or professional mistakes. Evaluation of the child protection systems in the various jurisdictions involved analyzing whether laws and practice comply with federal legal requirements (like the Adoption and Safe Families Act; ASFA).[5] Research results provided practical considerations for each jurisdiction, identifying policies and practices that were working well and those that required further discussion and adjustment.

UNDERSTANDING AND EVALUATING THE ROLE OF THE COURT IN CHILD PROTECTION CASES

Research findings emphasized that evaluation of the child protection system must include an analysis of the role and effectiveness of the dependency court system (the court with civil jurisdiction over child abuse and neglect cases). The role of the court in the child protection system is relatively new and constantly evolving, creating challenges in evaluation.

The local child protection agency is often viewed as central to the child protection system and perceived as operating autonomously with minimal accountability. For purposes of this article, "Department" refers to the local agency that provides child protection services, investigation, and case management. The child protection *system*, as the term is used in this article, is comprised of multiple entities (the department, health, law enforcement, etc.) which interact with families with overall case oversight coming from the dependency court.

The role of the court in child protection cases is critical, but the involvement of the court is often understated, partly because the court's role has evolved only in the last 20 years. As recently as the 1970s, juvenile and family courts were expected only to determine whether a child had been abused or neglected and, if so, whether the child(ren) needed to be removed from their homes. In the past, court involvement in cases was often a "rubber stamp" for department recommendations and plans. However, federal legislation enacted in the 1980s and 1990s increased the responsibilities and requirements of the legal system and judiciary in child protection cases. As a result, judicial oversight of dependency cases has increased. In essence, the child protection system is still evolving from a system "run" by the department into a larger system with multiple entities required by law to be held accountable by the court.

The relative newness of court involvement in child abuse and neglect cases has resulted in a child protection system where stakeholders operate with a mix of formal and informal practices that often conflict with each other, creating unintended consequences for children and parents. In general, dependency court judges are responsible for ensuring that the child's best interests are met and that a safe, permanent, and stable home is secured for each child coming before them. Among other things, this responsibility gives them the authority to evaluate the reasonableness of services provided to families; question the amount of visitation requested; inquire about the safety of a child's placement; request the child be present in court; and ensure that all stakeholders comply with procedural safeguards.[6] The role of the dependency court in the child protection system creates a formal legal process. This process relies heavily on accountability measures that balance the responsibilities and duties of multiple entities with the constitutional and legal rights of parents and children.

RESEARCH METHODS UTILIZED

One size does not fit all when it comes to child protection system research because child protection systems operate differently from state to state and often county to county within states. Research methods varied depending on the needs of each jurisdiction. In general, the research methods employed were as follows:

- *Statutory and local rule review*: All projects included an analysis of statutes, rules, and policies that create and regulate the child protection system process and local practice.
- *Court observation*: Standardized court observation tools were developed based on the hearing structure for each jurisdiction. Court observation provided a unique opportunity to see firsthand the treatment of the parties, the thoroughness of the proceedings, and the evidence that is presented to support decisions that impact the well-being and safety of children and parents.
- *Site visits/interviews*: Site visits and interviews with multiple stakeholders working at various points in the child protection system were critical to understanding how a local child protection system implemented policies and procedures. Discussions and meetings with stakeholders helped in the development of appropriate data collection instruments and provided context and depth to research findings.

- *Case file review*: Standardized data collection instruments were developed using information from statutes, departmental and court policies and forms, interviews with stakeholders, and were based on the American Bar Association's Children and the Law section forms as used in court improvement projects across the country. Draft instruments were also reviewed and commented on by local stakeholders and local institutional review boards.
- *Surveys with clients and stakeholders*: Surveys were utilized to collect information regarding the experience of parents and, in particular, domestic violence victims who were navigating the child protection system. Surveys were also used to capture the stakeholder observations and opinions.

KEY FINDINGS AND CONSIDERATIONS IN CHILD PROTECTION SYSTEM EVALUATION

The highlights from the research presented here are examples of some of the key points in case flow management, where specific system policies or procedures were found to impact the management of cases. Data demonstrate that some of these procedures affected how well-being and safety decisions were made for children and domestic violence victims. Data results presented here are limited due to space considerations for this article. Each jurisdiction's results and targeted strategies developed can be found in detailed reports.

The research focused on examining the "front-end" of how cases are managed as they move through the child protection system to identify what procedural gaps and challenges exist overall and what impact these gaps and challenges have on children exposed to violence and families experiencing domestic violence (see Figure 1).

EVALUATING KEY DEMOGRAPHIC DATA

Collecting demographic data is important to assist jurisdictions in determining whether the child protection system is documenting relevant information regarding children, like age and ethnicity. Collecting the age of the child involved with the child protection system is also critical in evaluating whether the system is considering age in (a) addressing benchmarks for physical health, mental health, and the educational needs of the child, and (b) allocating appropriate prevention and early intervention

FIGURE 1. Chart of the Child Protection System – "Front-End Process".

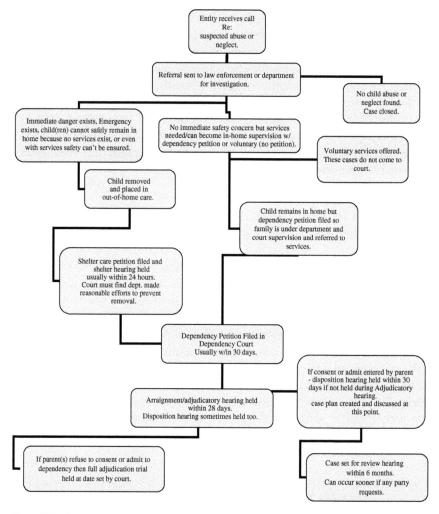

Note. This flow chart represents what generally happens when a child and parent(s) case comes into contact with the child protection system. The research design evaluated how practices utilized by various entities affected the management of cases flowing through this system.

resources relevant to particular age groups predominant in dependency cases. Results from the research sites indicate that not less than 50% of all child protection cases involve children in the infant-6 age group. Specifically in one jurisdiction, children age 6 and under accounted for

67.6% (n = 94 of 139) of all cases. Children age 3 and under accounted for 47.5% (n = 66 of 139) of all cases. These statistics demonstrate the large number of very young children who are involved in the child protection system and exposed to violence and the need for developmentally appropriate services and case planning.

EVALUATION OF THE DEPARTMENT'S PRIOR CONTACT WITH FAMILIES

Oftentimes, the department has had previous contact with parents and children that sometimes involves referral to services. For example, if a child abuse or neglect referral is made and the child is not in immediate danger, the department can refer a family to various supports and services to help prevent the need for child removal or supervision from the dependency court. Results demonstrate the frequency with which the department has had some contact with the family *before* the most recent event that prompted the filing of the most current dependency petition: the department offered services to the family prior to removing a child or filing a petition in approximately 50% of cases reviewed in multiple jurisdictions (n = 158 of 314).

Federal law requires departments to demonstrate that reasonable efforts have been made to provide assistance and services to prevent the unnecessary removal of a child from his/her home and make it possible for a child who has been placed in out-of-home care to be reunited with his/her family.[7] Reasonable effort determinations are made by the dependency court. The court made a specific finding of reasonable efforts in 70% of cases (n = 122 of 175) in one jurisdiction, but the lack of finding reasonable efforts in the other 30% of cases did not result in the case being dismissed or for any action to be taken toward the department.

EVALUATING THE REMOVAL OF CHILDREN

The Precipitating Event

The precipitating event is the factor that the investigative authority states as the predominant reason that warrants the immediate (emergency) removal of child(ren) from their primary caregiver. This information can be found on department investigation reports, but is most commonly found in the shelter care petition submitted to the dependency court. Other factors could also be present at the time of removal, but one particular event made the situation emergent and required immediate removal. The category of precipitating events utilized in the research projects generally mirrored the statutory allegations that permit the department and court to intervene in each jurisdiction. Collecting data on the precipitating event showed whether children were being removed primarily because they were witnesses to domestic violence. Children were removed from their primary caregiver in 62% of the cases reviewed in multiple jurisdictions (n = 195 of 314). In one jurisdiction (N = 139 cases), the events that precipitated removal of children included domestic violence (31.7%), child physical abuse (23.0%), drug/alcohol abuse (18.7%), mental health issues (12.9%), child neglect (9.4%), and criminal activity (4.3%). In this jurisdiction, the percentage of removals or petition filings based on domestic violence as the precipitating event promoted discussion regarding how domestic violence is identified, how the lethality of the domestic violence is assessed, and allowed for further data collection on the factors that generally co-occurred with domestic violence. In another jurisdiction (N = 97 cases involving domestic violence), co-occurring factors included mental health issues (30.9%), substance abuse (73.2%), child abuse (16.5%), and child neglect (8.2%). In another jurisdiction (N = 220 files reviewed), co-occurring factors included substance abuse (72% of mothers and 76% of fathers), mental health issues (48% of mothers and 12% of fathers), and criminal history (64% of mothers and 100% of fathers).

Placement Data

Collecting data regarding where children are placed after they are removed from their primary caregiver allows for a closer evaluation of placement decisions and their effect on children. Table 1 demonstrates data regarding the placement location of the children after removal as it correlates to the precipitating event that prompted the removal. When domestic violence was a factor contributing to the decision to file a dependency petition in some jurisdictions, data revealed that the child was sometimes placed with a spouse or relative with a history of domestic violence or a history of minimizing the ongoing domestic violence. This type of finding would indicate an area in case management requiring further scrutiny. Procedures and polices should ensure that placements for children are safe and require the court to ask questions of the department regarding how they investigated the new placement.

In cases where domestic violence is a factor, placement with the other parent or the batterer's relatives requires even closer scrutiny by the court and stakeholders to determine if this placement will actually: increase

TABLE 1. Placement location after removal (N = 105)

Precipitating Event	With Other, Mother	With Other, Father	With Relatives	Foster Care	"Department Custody"[a]	Total
Domestic violence	1	3	15	4	4	27
Mental health	0	0	8	1	7	16
Criminal activity	0	0	3	1	2	6
Drug use	0	1	13	2	6	22
Physical abuse	0	3	11	3	5	22
Other neglect	0	1	5	4	2	12
Total	1	8	55	15	26	105

[a]The Department Custody category represents those children in department custody whose location could not be determined from court records.

safety concerns for the child; aide the batterer in continuing the abuse; or elevate the risk of violence for the victim-parent and child. The court should closely scrutinize cases where the out-of-home placement is the other parent who may be "estranged" from the victim-parent and examine any relevant divorce or child custody orders to ensure that placement of the child does not violate an already existing court order.

EVALUATING THE DEPENDENCY PETITION

The dependency petition becomes the foundational pleading of the dependency court process and should contain critical information. Petitions in all four jurisdictions lacked clear information regarding why the parent(s) should be under the jurisdictions of the court and the specific facts that brought the case to the attention of the department. Stakeholders discussed the need to create petitions that contain case-specific allegations so that it is easier for the parent to understand why they are under the jurisdiction of the dependency court and how it relates to subsequent case planning. Petitions also need to provide enough detailed information to justify the department and court choices for treatment and services.

ADJUDICATION HEARING EVALUATION

Adjudication hearings are held unless the petition is withdrawn prior to the hearing date. Data should be collected regarding when an adjudication or arraignment takes place to ensure that practice is in compliance with the time period outlined in statute. Compliance with statutory timelines can create a better opportunity for children to reach permanency and for the state to comply with ASFA. However, ASFA also requires that timelines be balanced with protecting the safety and well-being of the child. Strict adherence to timelines should not take the place of properly determining what is in the best interests of the child. Combined statistics from two jurisdictions indicate that 82% of the 212 cases that went to an adjudication hearing were adjudicated based on the parent(s) consent without the presentation of testimony or evidence. In addition, in the 582 case files reviewed in all four jurisdictions little information could be found regarding what took place at hearings. Many of the court orders merely stated the next hearing date and did not indicate the new or standing orders of the court.

When data demonstrate that adjudication is taking place in the majority of cases based on consent, questions should be raised regarding whether all the checks and balances afforded in this legal process are being implemented. Areas to consider evaluating more closely include: due process issues, notice issues, and parent representation issues. Consider whether the court is requiring "hard" evidence in the form of paperwork, assessments, and testimony to support the department's assertions (petition allegations) regarding the presenting problems in the family. For example, stating that a parent has a "domestic violence history" without referring to supporting evidence creates the potential for the development of inappropriate case plans.

EVALUATING THE SYSTEM EXPERIENCE OF PARENTS AND CHILDREN EXPOSED TO DOMESTIC VIOLENCE

When multiple co-occurring factors are present and one of them is domestic violence, a closer assessment by the child protection system is required. The safety and well-being of children exposed to violence needs proper assessment so the court can make appropriate decisions regarding their welfare. Results indicate that cases existed where children who witnessed the domestic violence were removed from their families, not solely because they witnessed violence but due to the imminent danger to their physical and emotional health posed by a combination of all the presenting risk factors and the nonviability of other solutions.

The increased awareness of the potential for children exposed to domestic violence to suffer harmful effects has increased the amount of child protection cases that identify domestic violence as a relevant factor. Identification of domestic violence in child protection cases emphasizes the importance of evaluating whether the child protection system process has evolved to appropriately address intervention and treatment *after* the identification occurs.

After reviewing cases in multiple jurisdictions, data indicate that the removal of children usually occurs when there are multiple risk factors and dangers to the children that cannot be immediately mitigated. Children were rarely removed solely for witnessing an incident of domestic violence; however, research did indicate that some policies and procedures were inadequate to properly address the safety and well-being of all families, which posed a risk of disproportionately impacting parent(s) and children experiencing domestic violence because their safety and well-being issues can be more complex.

Victim Data from Dependency Court Files

Data results from the jurisdictions emphasized the need for improvement in policies and procedures to increase the accuracy of identification of the victim and batterer in the family. In the cases studied, proper identification at the beginning of the case strongly influenced whether appropriate safety measures were put into place and services ordered for the victim-parent, the batterer, and the child witnesses. In all four jurisdictions, it appeared that identifying which parent was the victim and which was the batterer was not consistently or accurately done. In 314 cases reviewed in multiple jurisdictions, 139 cases identified domestic violence as a factor; of these 139 cases, the mother was identified as the victim in 65% ($n = 90$) of cases and the father or a paramour were identified as the victim in 35% ($n = 49$) of cases. The mother, father, and a significant other were also identified as the batterer in the same case in 9% ($n = 13$) of cases. Beyond the obvious and critical safety concerns that may be ignored when a victim is not appropriately identified, not accurately identifying the victim also creates problems in developing an appropriate case plan for service (i.e., support services versus anger management) and developing appropriate orders for placement and visitation (i.e., removing the child from victim-parent and only allowing supervised visitation).

Table 2 presents the percentage of cases where supervised visits were ordered per precipitating factor in one jurisdiction. In this jurisdiction, the high percentage of supervised visitation for the mother in domestic violence situations required stakeholders to take a closer look at whether department

TABLE 2. Percentage of cases where supervised visits ordered per precipitating factor in one jurisdiction (N = 81)

Supervised Visits Ordered in Case Plan	Domestic Violence	Mental Health	Other Criminal Activity	Substance Abuse	Child Abuse	Child Neglect
Father	33.3%	11.1%	6.2%	14.8%	22.2%	12.4%
Mother	26.6%	15.2%	6.3%	18.9%	20.3%	12.7%

recommendations regarding supervised visitation were subjective or objective. Discussions resulted in stakeholders re-evaluating the effectiveness of the current supervised visitation policies and procedures. Many stakeholders did not realize that ordered supervised visitation without clear orders on where and how often it was to take place was creating situations where many parents did not see their children for weeks or months.

Data collected from the department and court files and from victim-parent surveys provided findings on how often a victim-parent attempted to obtain a restraining order/injunction (whether told to or not), whether a restraining order/injunction was granted, whether the victim-parent requested that the restraining order/injunction or no contact order be dropped, and whether the department requested that the victim get a domestic violence restraining order/injunction. Evaluation also included collecting data to determine the percentage of victim-parents who are arrested to determine if victim-parents are being inappropriately identified as a co-batterer; this occurred in 19% ($n = 27$ of 143) of cases. Stakeholders in all four jurisdictions were surprised that although domestic violence was identified, critical information regarding how the system offered or provided adequate safety constructs for the victim-parents was not well documented.

The victim-parent survey collected information that most likely would not be contained in a court or department case file (e.g., whether the victim-parent was told to separate from the batterer by department; whether the department assisted the victim-parent in accomplishing the separation; or whether the victim-parent was told by the department that their child might be taken away from them if they did not take steps to protect themselves from the batterer). The results showed that victim-parents "experience" with the department regarding the domestic violence was largely dependent on the investigator or caseworker they were assigned and that this department professional believed they were a victim and supported their safety concerns. The involvement and support that local domestic violence professionals provided the victim-parent was also a critical factor in whether they felt supported in the child protection system.

Capturing the Domestic Violence History and Types of Domestic Violence

The purpose of collecting data on parents' domestic violence history is two-fold. First, it is used to identify whether the child protection system is actively identifying cases with domestic violence. Second, it is used to identify how domestic violence is captured as a presenting factor in a current case. Assessing how the system is identifying a history of domestic violence is significant because just stating the term "domestic violence history" in court documents without proper supporting information can lead to inappropriate decisions in the case. Screening tools should ask questions which help stakeholders distinguish between cases with current domestic violence incidents with immediate safety and well-being concerns versus incidents that happened years ago and the domestic violence is no longer a prevalent problem in the family.

In one jurisdiction, the domestic violence incident histories in 96 cases were recorded as follows: present domestic violence (57.3%); domestic violence within 1 year (15.6%); domestic violence within 1–2 years (11.5%); and domestic violence within 2 or more years (6.3%). In 9.4% of cases, a domestic violence experience was mentioned, but whether the domestic violence occurred currently or in the past could not be determined. Data were collected by reviewing a variety of documents in the files. No report existed in the case files that answered the incident history questions directly.

The nature and severity of domestic violence varies from victim to victim, as does the impact of the violence on the victim. Determining the nature and severity of the violence assists the department and the court in determining appropriate services and significantly impacts lethality and safety assessments. Appropriate assessments should also consider other safety constructs, such as the risk of violence in the future, the child's degree of exposure and resilience, the victim's resilience and ability to protect the child, the presence of protective factors in the immediate and extended family, and available support from the community.[8]

The nature and severity of the domestic violence was captured using categories of violence and behavior and by reviewing multiple records in the case files. No document existed in any jurisdiction that recorded the information consistently or in a standardized form. More than one category could be marked for each of 110 cases in the following results from multiple jurisdictions: verbal argument (66.4%); pushing/shoving/no marks (75.4%); physical abuse (60%); kidnapping/false imprisonment (12.7%); sexual assault: (0.04%); emotional/verbal abuse (0.08%); and intimidation/threats (28.2%).

Data were collected to demonstrate the frequency of various events in the child protection system with respect to how domestic violence cases were managed ($N = 44$). Over 68% had previous contact with child protection services, 56.8% received services prior to removal, 18.2% had a prior petition, and in 61.4% of cases, a child had been removed. Victim-parent survey results showed that in cases in which domestic violence was present but was not the precipitating event, children were removed in 50% of cases ($N = 92$ children). Data results from the case file review were similar to the experience of victim-parents surveyed, in that roughly half of all children were removed from the victim-parent experiencing domestic violence; however, more than half of these cases also had services offered to them before the removal occurred as well as other co-occurring factors.

The Domestic Violence Batterer

Accurate identification of the domestic violence batterer is critical for the child protection system, but data demonstrate that when domestic violence is identified by the system, management of the batterer is not a priority. In cases that actually contained information about the batterer, results showed that the batterer: was arrested in 48.3% of cases ($n = 69$ of 143); was removed from the home by law enforcement or through the filing of an injunction or no contact order in 43.4% of cases ($n = 62$ of 143); had subsequently returned home prior to completion of the case plan in 29.5% of cases ($n = 28$ of 96); was criminally charged in 30.8% of cases ($n = 44$ of 143); or was referred to batterer appropriate services in 44.8% of cases ($n = 43$ of 96).

When information on the batterer could be found, these queries provided an objective perspective on whether the child protection system was holding the batterer accountable. Comparing these percentages with the victim-parent data provided an objective analysis as to whether the child protection system process treats the victim-parent and the batterer-parent fairly and appropriately with respect to the domestic violence factor. Data from the jurisdictions indicate that the batterer is often viewed as secondary in the dependency case and the victim is placed in the primary role as adequate or inadequate caregiver to the child. Oftentimes, the batterer, if identified, was not arrested or held accountable by the criminal (i.e., charges, jail) or civil legal systems (i.e., injunctions) or the department (i.e., supervised visitation, batterer appropriate services).

CHILD WITNESSES TO DOMESTIC VIOLENCE

Data on the frequency of exposure to domestic violence for children in the child protection system was collected from a variety of sources in the department and court files. The data collected at the project sites ranged from stakeholders asking no questions of the child to a child's experience being detailed in reports. In multiple jurisdictions, court and department file data indicate that the child witnessed the domestic violence in 65.5% of cases ($n = 114$ of 174) and that the child received physical injuries during a domestic violence incident in 16.2% of the cases ($n = 23$ of 142). These figures might be higher if this critical information was consistently collected in a uniform manner.

For a system presumably designed to "protect children," the lack of consistent information in the files regarding the safety and well-being of children, including the degree to which they have been exposed to violence, was alarming. However, it creates an opportunity for stakeholders to re-evaluate the focus of the child protection system and to improve assessment and documentation of children's needs. Stakeholder perceptions on the purpose of the child protection system and the goals for the families varied depending on their system profession. It is critical for stakeholders to discuss how best to balance the needs and requirements of the parents, while addressing the well-being and safety concerns of the child(ren).

LESSONS LEARNED

The practical system-wide assessments that were conducted allowed jurisdictions to identify practices that increase fragmentation and negative outcomes. This targeted identification permitted them to strategically begin to correct practice. Stakeholders agreed that the objective data on how their particular child protection system was operating helped them have: an improved understanding of the practices that are within the control of each particular agency or entity and those that are not; a working knowledge of the roles and responsibilities of each agency or entity; and an understanding of the laws, policies, and procedures that provide the framework for the system process.

Stakeholders were invested in the results because they were consulted throughout the assessment and assisted in interpreting the results. How research methods were developed and implemented was as important as the results. Many stakeholders commented that they appreciated that the assessment was conducted by an objective professional from outside the community who demonstrated a working knowledge of the challenges faced by legal, social service, and domestic violence professionals. They stressed the importance of having an evaluator that took the time to understand how the child protection system functioned in *their* jurisdiction and community. Research was conducted with limited resources and staff, but the intense and focused nature of the projects allowed for comprehensive results from multiple sources.

Overall, stakeholders acknowledged that (a) revising practices using data is likely to be wiser than when they are developed based solely on anecdotal experiences with the system; (b) the data could be used to define a problem as opposed to bargaining over the perceived cause of the problem; and (c) unlike arbitrary or anecdotal perceptions, data sometimes reveal a procedural gap that is directly on point and accepted by all as in need of repair.

Ultimately, the expectation is that solutions created within this assessment framework will increase stakeholders' abilities to appropriately identify, evaluate, and assist families within the larger context of the child protection system. In cases where domestic violence is a primary factor, the research can improve those practices that are identified as disproportionately and negatively impacting the safety and well-being of these families. The assessments were successful in establishing a flexible research design that examined practice within a continuum as opposed to examining practices within the isolation of only one entity, agency, or department. As child protection systems evolve, the insight gained from research can assist professionals in improving practice with the ultimate goal of improving outcomes for all children and their families.

NOTES

1. Carlson, B. E. (2000). Children exposed to intimate partner violence: Research findings and implications for interventions. *Trauma, Violence and Abuse, 1*(4), 321–340.

2. Appel, A. E., & Holden, G. W. (1998). The co-occurrence of spouse and physical child abuse: A review and appraisal. *Journal of Family Psychology, 12*(4), 578–599.

3. Child Information Gateway Fact Sheet. (2007). 2–3: www.childwelfare.gov/pubs/factsheets/domestic violence.cfm

4. See Kracke and Cohen (2008, this issue) for a comprehensive discussion of the Safe Start Initiative. Kracke, K., & Cohen, E. (2008). The Safe Start Initiative: Building and disseminating knowledge to support children exposed to violence. *Journal of Emotional Abuse, 8*(1/2), 155–174.

5. *Adoption and Safe Families Act of 1997* (P.L. 105–89).

6. National Council of Juvenile and Family Court Judges. (1995). *Resource guidelines: Improving court practice in child abuse and neglect cases.* Reno, NV: Author. Available from http://www.ncjfcj.org/content/blogcategory/369/438/

7. Beginning with the Adoption Assistance and Child Welfare Act of 1980 (P.L. 96–272).

8. National Council of Juvenile and Family Court Judges (NCJFCJ). (1999). *Effective intervention in domestic violence & child maltreatment cases: Guidelines for policy and practice.* Commonly referred to as the "Greenbook," p. 64.

Children Exposed to Violence at School: An Evidence-based Intervention Agenda for the "Real" Bullying Problem

Samuel Y. Song
Karen Callan Stoiber

Children are frequently exposed to violence in the school setting. Although the level of school violence has been declining during the last decade (U.S. Secret Service & U.S. Department of Education, 2002), it remains a pernicious problem that affects the health and well-being of all students (Farrell, Meyer, Kung, & Sullivan, 2001). The most prevalent type of school violence is bullying. Bullying has been referred to as peer abuse because it shares certain characteristics that are similar to other forms of abuse and maltreatment. These characteristics include: hurtful behavior that is physical, verbal, emotional, or social in nature; the behavior is repetitive over time or chronic; and there is a power differential in which the victims of bullying are unable to adequately defend themselves against it or to make it stop (Olweus, 1991).

Bullying can result in severe psychological, academic, and physical harm to the victim, as well as adverse outcomes for the perpetrator and peers who witness it (Nishina, Juvonen, & Witkow, 2005; O'Connell, Pepler, & Craig, 1999). Based on student reports and observations on playgrounds, bullying is widespread at both the elementary and high school level (Flannery, Wester, & Singer, 2004; Frey et al., 2005b). Nansel et al. (2001) found that approximately 1 out of every 5 children is chronically bullied. Rates for witnessing bullying are higher, with Flannery et al. (2004) finding almost 9 of 10 high-school students reported witnessing someone being hit, slapped, or punched at school. Four percent of school students reported that they had missed school within the last 30 days because they feared being intimidated or bullied (Kann et al., 1998). These findings are alarming as bullying seems not only to undermine a child's fundamental right to learn in a safe school environment (e.g., Schwartz, Gorman, Nakamoto, & Toblin, 2005) but can potentially result in irreparable harm (Nishina et al., 2005).

At a societal level, the impact of bullying may be more devastating: A retrospective study by the U.S. Secret Service and the Department of Education (2002) examining school shootings between 1974–2000 found that 71% of the school shooters ($N = 29$) were victims of chronic bullying. Indeed, bullying has been identified recently as the primary target for prevention and intervention of more severe violent acts that occur in schools (Skiba et al., 2006). Researchers have responded to the prevalence and problems of bullying by designing comprehensive school-based programs aimed at altering peer aggression at multiple levels within the school ecology (Swearer & Doll, 2001). However, preventing bullying effectively has been challenging for primarily two reasons. First, bullying is difficult to address due to its complex nature and the level of coordination required for effective implementation of comprehensive intervention strategies at the individual, classroom, and school level. Second, the state-of-the-science is equivocal in the area of effective bullying prevention and intervention (i.e., evidence-based interventions (EBIs)), as most evaluations of whole school anti-bullying programs have yielded nonsignificant results (Smith, Schneider, Smith, & Ananiadou, 2004).

In this article, our purpose is to advance the field of children exposed to violence by proposing a broader conceptualization of the school bullying problem and a model for how to address it. The extant bullying prevention and intervention literature is reviewed with these aims: (a) examine the challenge of *effective* school bullying prevention and intervention more fully; and (b) propose an EBI agenda that focuses on the problem of bullying in schools.

CHALLENGES TO EFFECTIVE BULLYING PREVENTION

Ecological Phenomenon

School bullying involves much more than the two roles of bully and victim; bullying involves the whole school. Therefore, it is best viewed as an ecological phenomenon in which it emerges from social, physical, institutional, and community environments as well as the individual characteristics of the youth involved (Swearer & Doll, 2001). Within this ecological framework, the disposition in the individual (e.g., limited social competencies, negative attributions, poor emotion regulation skills) interacts with the social environment (e.g., peer relationships, class rules, teacher behaviors, school culture) to foster bullying behavior (Bronfenbrenner, 1979; Pianta & Walsh, 1996). Various ecological factors can have a powerful influence on school bullying by either encouraging or maintaining its occurrence (Doll, Song, & Siemers, 2002; Hirschstrein, Edstrom, Frey, Snell, & MacKenzie, 2007; Orpinas & Horne, 2006). These researchers have documented several important ecological factors to consider, including teachers' implementation of bullying prevention lessons, teacher coaching of students involved in bullying, teacher beliefs about bullying, and victim and peer responses to bullying.

A review of research on ecological factors affecting bullying indicates several interesting findings. First, qualitative aspects of intervention programs, including the degree to which teachers incorporate interactive instructional techniques such as role playing and peer coaching, has been associated with reduced aggression among students (Conduct Problems Prevention Research Group, 1999). This finding regarding the quality of teacher delivery is an important one as teachers implementing bullying prevention programs report much lower use of role plays than of more didactic teacher-led activities (Kallestad & Olweus, 2003). Thus it appears teachers who implement bullying prevention may omit the more effective strategies of engaging students in explicit skill rehearsal and student-generated solutions to bullying problems. This emphasis on "telling" students how to behave is unfortunate as such didactic methods do not likely lead to a student appropriately asserting oneself during a conflict (Hirschstein et al., 2007).

Second, teachers and school personnel may not respond in ways that discourage bullying, but rather may contribute to it through inaction (Boulton & Underwood, 1992; Hoover, Oliver, & Hazler, 1992; Olweus, 1991; Twemlow et al., 2001). School adults intervene at low rates despite teacher reports of higher intervention (Craig & Pepler, 1997; Leff, Kupersmidt, Patterson, & Power, 1999). Teacher inaction during bullying episodes may be due to pro-bullying beliefs and limited knowledge about bullying. Over 90% of teachers acknowledged that bullying occurred in the classroom but minimized it, while 25% believed it was helpful to ignore it (Stephenson & Smith, 1989). Third, peers also tend not to intervene during bullying episodes despite being present 85% of the time (Craig & Pepler, 1997; Naylor & Cowie, 1999). Some peers have actively joined in the bullying, while others have encouraged bullying by watching, laughing, or remaining silent (Craig & Pepler, 1997; Naylor & Cowie, 1999; Salmivalli, Lagerspetz, Bjorkvist, Osterman, & Kaukianen, 1996). Finally, within this bullying-encouraging context, it should not be surprising to learn that victims also do not seek help from others. Children who are bullied may also encourage bullying by not telling teachers or adults about their difficulties (Pepler, Craig, Ziegler, & Charach, 1994). This may be due to fear of retaliation from the bully or because they perceived adults as inept, uncaring, or unable to protect them (Pepler et al., 1994).

To summarize, bullying is extremely complex and involves multiple factors within the school ecology that work together to encourage and maintain bullying rather than discouraging it. How can schools address these powerful ecological factors related to bullying?

The Uneasy State-of-the-Science

In response to the bullying epidemic, school district adoption of anti-bullying policies for the establishment of bullying prevention and intervention strategies is increasing across the country (Limber & Small, 2003). It should be no surprise that most practitioners and researchers agree that there is an urgent need for practices proven to banish bullying behaviors in school settings, and that such practices should be research-based. Although intervention research in general has been evident since the early 1900s, the interest in translating research findings into effective instructional and intervention practices has been particularly invigorated with the EBI movement (Kratochwill, 2006; Shavelson & Towne, 2002; Stoiber & Kratochwill, 2000, 2002a, 2002b). Thus, the interest in developing EBIs to counter bullying necessarily points to the desire for interventions that can be effectively applied in real school settings.

Despite well-established literature on what bullying is and its effects at the individual, classroom, and school level, there exists limited empirical evidence of the effectiveness of bullying intervention programs. In particular, there is a dearth of peer-reviewed research on these programs. Without well-designed research, we cannot move forward in determining what bullying interventions work, and moreover, what conditions are necessary for optimal outcomes to be achieved. Hence, there is a clear need not only for anti-bullying intervention programs, but for high quality intervention studies that examine essential program dimensions and components.

Just as researchers have criticized the quantity and quality of research in important areas affecting student educational outcomes, such as reading (Troia, 1999), early childhood (Snyder, Thompson, McLean, & Smith, 2002), emotional disturbance (Mooney, Epstein, Reid, & Nelson, 2003), and special education (Seethaler & Fuchs, 2005), we believe there is an urgent need to establish an evidence base in the area of bullying interventions. The following criteria have been considered pertinent in determining effectiveness of instructional interventions:

a. used an experimental and/or quasi-experimental design;
b. occurred for a reasonable length of time;
c. incorporated multiple outcome measures;
d. collected post-intervention as well as follow-up data after a specified period of time subsequent to program implementation;
e. assessed treatment integrity (i.e., degree to which intervention was implemented as intended);

f. employed appropriate statistical methods;
g. had a sufficient sample size to measure effects;
h. showed significant positive effects on appropriate outcomes, such as improved school climate or school safety (Stoiber & Waas, 2002).

Thus for a bullying intervention strategy to be considered "evidence-based" or "effective," it should be supported by research meeting-specified criteria. For this to occur, however, considerable changes in the characteristics of bullying intervention research are indicated. In the interest of space, we highlight the primary concerns.

A number of bullying interventions have been developed to alter the frequency and degree of bullying behavior, with the aim of improving student safety and academic, health, and mental health functioning (Flannery et al., 2004; Hirschstein et al., 2007). Most of these bullying intervention approaches are comprehensive, utilizing multiple components to target a broad range of bully, victim, and bystander decisions and behaviors throughout the "whole school." Such comprehensive, whole-school bullying intervention programs are often viewed as most efficacious, with one program reporting a significant reduction of bullying by 50% (Olweus, Limber, & Mihalic, 1999). However, recent meta-analyses of whole-school bullying intervention research have found that many replication studies have no beneficial effect, and surprisingly some have a negative effect on bullying (Smith et al., 2004). The primary reason for these mixed results was the poor quality of intervention implementation (also referred to as feasibility of an intervention, intervention fidelity, or treatment integrity). Indeed, in a recent comprehensive examination of education intervention studies, treatment integrity was measured less than 15% of the time (Gresham, MacMillan, Beebe-Frankenberger, & Bocian, 2000; Snyder et al., 2002; Wolery & Garfinkle, 2002). Interestingly, in the study conducted by Smith and colleagues (2004), greater effects were shown in the bullying intervention studies where intervention fidelity was addressed; specifically, they found a greater reduction in student-reported victimization. When measurement of intervention fidelity has occurred, measurement has typically focused on teacher didactic or "talk and tell" features. The importance of addressing intervention fidelity in intervention research cannot be understated. Stoiber and Kratochwill (2002a) conclude that perhaps the greatest obstacles to establishing EBIs pertains to the interrelated issues of acceptance, feasibility, and sustainability: acceptability is the degree to which consumers find the intervention procedures and outcomes acceptable in their daily lives; feasibility is the degree to which intervention components can be implemented in naturalistic contexts; and sustainability is the extent to which the intervention can be maintained without support from external agents.

The real life issues of acceptance, feasibility, and sustainability may also contribute to another limitation in the current bullying intervention literature: the failure of researchers to collect follow-up data. Whereas typical school-and classroom-based bullying interventions would seemingly need to occur over a substantial period of time to produce meaningful and long-term effects, little work to date has examined effects beyond 1 year (Hirschstein et al., 2007) and most assess effects immediately following the intervention (Smith et al., 2004). Regarding issues of acceptability, feasibility, and sustainability, the lack of long-term outcome research is likely due to the fact that teachers and administrators typically resist the random assignment of students to classrooms for experimental purposes, especially for an extended period of time. School administrators typically assess the cost-benefit ratio to make sure that the intervention is both cost-effective and practical to implement. For example, what are the costs with regard to materials, time, and training? For schools and staff to "buy in" to bullying intervention programs, such costs must be balanced against the expected "payoffs" of the intervention. As noted earlier, teachers often "miss" incidences of bullying, and thus may underestimate the degree to which bullying is viewed as a problem "big enough" to require a comprehensive intervention approach.

Summary and the "Real" Bullying Problem

The fields of children exposed to violence, school violence prevention, and education are facing quite a complex dilemma in school bullying. There are two central challenges that make school bullying intervention difficult: addressing the numerous ecological factors that contribute to bullying and improving the real-world feasibility of comprehensive bullying intervention programs in schools. Clearly, the problem of school bullying is broader than simply the negative outcomes associated with it. The "real" bullying problem consists of the ecological factors that encourage and maintain bullying, which are compounded by the real-world challenge of improving intervention fidelity in existing school-based bullying intervention programs. In the next section, we propose an EBI agenda that focuses on the real bullying problem.

AN EVIDENCE-BASED INTERVENTION AGENDA FOR ADDRESSING THE REAL BULLYING PROBLEM

Addressing the ecological complexity of the bullying phenomenon and the real-life complexity of intervention research and practice requires innovation, conceptually and practically. Based on extant theory and research, this section discusses the rationale for an innovative conceptual framework for effective school bullying prevention focusing on the critical processes that reduce bullying—the protective peer ecology. First, the peer ecology is introduced and the protective peer ecology is discussed with the rationale for its importance. Next, the integration of the protective peer ecology framework within existing school practices is proposed with an illustration. Finally, a model for innovative bullying intervention practice is presented.

Protective Peer Ecology Conceptual Framework for Effective Bullying Prevention

From an ecological framework, peers are part of the microsystem, which is the immediate, proximal setting in which behavior unfolds and is an essential context for development. "The peer ecology is that part of a children's microsystem that involves children interacting with, influencing, and socializing one another. Peer ecologies do not include adults, but can affect and be affected by them" (Rodkin & Hodges, 2003, p. 384).

The peer ecology may be the most influential context for bullying prevention (Song, 2006; Song, Doll, Swearer, & Johnsen, 2005; Song, Doll, Swearer, Johnsen, & Siegel, in press) and as such may be the best target for bullying prevention. Peers can help correct the inherent power imbalance between bullies and victims and can help address the pro-bullying school environments effectively (i.e., inaction of school personnel). For example, peers can protect one another from bullying more effectively than adult school personnel because peers are typically present during the majority of bullying interactions, and they can detect even the covert occurrences of bullying (e.g., Craig & Pepler, 1997). Victims of bullying may also be more likely to come to a peer for help and support instead of school personnel.

Finally, peers are a naturally existing school resource that may substantially reduce intervention implementation burdens for schools, thereby addressing the real-world challenges for effective prevention. This idea may be the most compelling reason to focus on peers. Indeed, experts in EBIs have advocated for more research focusing on the identification of the critical mechanisms that lead to improved outcomes (Hoagwood & Olin, 2002). Once identified, innovative interventions can be developed that target the critical mechanisms producing streamlined yet powerful interventions (Kazdin, 2001; Schoenwald & Hoagwood, 2001; Weersing & Weisz, 2002; Weisz, 2000). These streamlined programs are likely to be more feasible to implement and thus more effective. Further research needs to focus on the peer ecology and the identification of the critical peer processes that lead to reduced bullying.

Protective Peer Ecology

To guide the investigation of critical processes within the peer ecology, the idea of a protective peer ecology is helpful (Song, 2006; Song et al., 2005, in press). A protective peer ecology refers to the aspects of children's interactions with one another that serve as a shield against internal or external sources of stress. Rodkin and Hodges (2003) explained that peer ecologies include social structures that organize children's behavior horizontally and vertically. Horizontal structure includes numerous and diverse social relationships, which provide multiple paths for children to enjoy social support. Examples include dyadic friendships, peer groups, and enemy relationships. Vertical structure of peer ecologies refers to social power, social status, and the consequent degree of influence. Some children have more power in the peer group and are more valued than other children.

In support of the protective peer ecology, research has convincingly demonstrated that positive peer affiliations (i.e., having a friend, number of friendships, peer acceptance) are significantly related to being bullied less (Hodges et al., 1997; Pellegrini et al., 1999). It has also been demonstrated that complex peer group dynamics had a strong influence on peer behaviors toward bullying (Cairns et al., 1995; Farmer et al., 2003). Other researchers have supported protection from friends by showing that having friends who are strong and aggressive was more important in being bullied less than having friends who lacked these characteristics (Hodges & Perry, 1999). Additional research has supported the importance of protection directly. These researchers found that protection provided by a best friend was the mechanism by which having a best friend was related to being bullied less over 1 year (Hodges et al., 1999). Finally, many bullying prevention researchers believe that peers who protect others are a critical mechanism for bullying prevention and have advocated for schools to create an "anti-bullying" culture among their students (Frey et al., 2005b; Olweus, Limber, & Mihalic, 1999).

To summarize, we have discussed the rationale for why the protective peer ecology is essential for effective bullying prevention. Theoretically, peers may be the best suited to address the complex ecological factors that encourage and maintain bullying in schools. On a practical level, mobilizing peers as interveners may ease implementation burdens on schools because peers are "already there." Finally, there is strong evidence supporting the importance of peers in reducing bullying, including general peer relation factors such as positive peer relationships and direct peer action to protect others from bullying, both of which are important in understanding a protective peer ecology against bullying.

Improved Implementation and Integration with Existing School Practices

The protective peer ecology framework is advantageous for effective school bullying prevention because interventions can specifically target this high priority area while still leading to important reductions in bullying. Protective peer ecological interventions may be more likely to be found acceptable by school personnel and implemented because they are more manageable compared to multi-component bullying programs, and better implementation should lead to increased sustainability of the intervention over time. Thus, achieving high implementation and sustainability will lead to better outcomes for children who are exposed to peer abuse.

Focusing on the protective peer ecology for bullying prevention will also produce less redundancy with other school intervention programs, which likely contributes to fewer implementation challenges in schools. For example, numerous schools are concerned with developing children socially and academically and have turned to prevention models that follow a three-tiered approach, such as school-wide positive behavior supports (PBS; Sugai & Horner, 2006). In addition to PBS, implementing another school-wide intervention program (e.g., a comprehensive bullying prevention program) may very well conflict directly with existing school resources. However, the protective peer ecology framework can and should be integrated into existing school-wide intervention programs like PBS, without being redundant and adding unnecessary intervention components. To illustrate more fully, Figure 1 depicts the protective peer ecology model; and later, we explain further how the protective peer ecology framework for bullying prevention might be integrated with the three-tiered PBS model.

FIGURE 1. Protective Peer Ecology Framework in Schools.

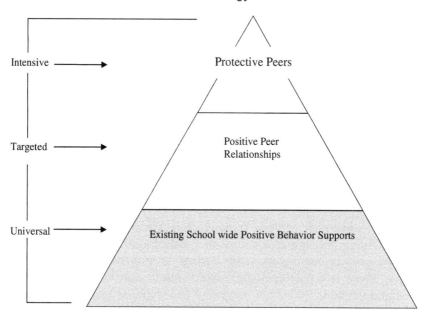

Universal Level

The first level is universal and consists of intervention components that are applied to all children. School- and classroom-wide interventions that include all school personnel across all settings are common. Bullying interventions that are also universal should be integrated into the already existing universal program. For example, school-wide PBS is already focusing on promoting positive behavior among all students, which includes disruptive and aggressive behaviors. The PBS intervention is simultaneously contributing to the reduction of bullying because bullying often grows from more typical aggressive behaviors (Doll et al., 2002). From a protective peer ecology framework, the only additional intervention strategy might consist of incorporating a focus on prosocial helping behaviors (especially during bullying episodes) and peer inclusion activities (e.g., rules like no one plays alone, no one eats alone; Doll, Zucker, & Brehm, 2004). Furthermore, teachers might also use traditional classroom management strategies to influence these important peer ecological factors that are related to less bullying. These strategies may be accomplished by tailoring existing PBS interventions rather than adding in a completely new intervention component.

Targeted Level

At a more targeted level, bullying interventions should focus on children who are at risk for bullying or who are exhibiting some precursory difficulties with bullying, either as the bully or victim. After identifying these children, teachers could be more deliberate about using prosocial helping behaviors and peer inclusion activities in their classrooms and on school grounds. For example, teachers could implement a peer helping intervention and make sure that these children are part of the intervention. Furthermore, teachers could ensure that these children are included during recess and lunch by implementing a recess activity that includes these students. For students at risk for being victims of bullying, peer support groups may be appropriate. Because of the potential for deviant peer influences, it is not recommended that students at risk for bullying others participate in group interventions (Dishion, McCord, & Poulin, 1999). Finally, another avenue for intervention would be to focus on children who encourage bullying and helping them develop empathy for victims of bullying.

Intensive Level

More intensive intervention is needed for children having greater difficulty with bullying others. Some recommended practices have been an individualized behavioral plan from a functional behavioral assessment (FBA) and individual counseling or therapy with these children. However, what has been missing from prior recommendations has been a focus on the victims. The assumption has been that focusing on the bully is sufficient. Although this may be true to a certain extent, it has been shown that victims of bullying are frequently bullied by other children (including the popular and well-adjusted children; Farmer et al., 2003) and in other settings (classrooms, grades). Therefore, if interventions do not address the victims, they may likely be bullied by other children at other times and in other settings.

Although FBA's and individual counseling can be tailored to victims, other interventions may be helpful. Group counseling might be used for chronic victims of bullying. Use of prosocial helping behaviors and peer inclusion activities might also be effective. For example, teachers could have prosocial and assertive children pair up with chronic victims of bullying as a peer buddy during potential bullying situations and try to incorporate the chronic victims of bullying into a peer group.

Evidence-Based Practice Model for Bullying Intervention

The protective peer ecology framework is helpful in conceptualizing targets for bullying intervention, which should inform the development of EBIs. Another issue having particular relevance for a bullying EBI agenda is recognition that different schools reflect diverse ecological and complex qualities, ones that often cannot be captured through the use of "traditional" laboratory-like procedures and methodologies. Bullying behavior has been shown to differ along the dimensions of age, race, economic levels, and community type. Higher levels of bullying behavior have been documented in the following demographic characteristics: (a) older students, (b) non-White students, (c) lower economic level students, and (d) urban school settings (Flannery et al., 2004). One bullying intervention program that incorporates several features considered necessary for meeting criteria of an EBI is the Steps to Respect Program (Committee on Children, 2001). Research by Frey, Hirschstein, Edstrom, and Snell (2005a, 2005b) on the Steps to Respect Program has incorporated an experimental design with randomized assignment of schools to treatment and multiple outcome indicators (self-report and observational measures). However, the evaluation of the Steps to Respect Program has occurred in suburban districts in the Pacific Northwest with a majority of Caucasian students (with Asian students as next most prevalent non-White group of students).

Given the fluctuating data on bullying incidence levels and differential response to bullying intervention strategies due to student economic backgrounds, ethnicity, and community setting (Flannery et al., 2004), broader application of programs such as the Steps to Respect Program in diverse schools and classrooms must occur before effective bullying strategies based on scientific principles and empirical data can be deduced. As such, we propose that practitioners function as researchers by applying data-based approaches for systematic planning, monitoring, and evaluating outcomes of their own service delivery in the area of bullying prevention and intervention. That is, due to noted limitations in the design and implementation of bullying prevention and intervention programs, there is a lack of evidence for using particular interventions with particular children in particular contexts (i.e., situated knowledge).

In adopting an evidence-based practice (EBP) model, school-based practitioners hold a central role in determining the effectiveness of bullying interventions in their own practice (Kratochwill, 2006; Stoiber & Kratochwill, 2002b; Stoiber, Lewis-Snyder, & Miller, 2005). For example, school-based consultants might promote teachers' use of goal attainment or other progress monitoring methods to determine whether selected anti-bullying strategies such as role playing "cool and calm" responses to bullying provocation and promoting good peer relations reduce the likelihood of victimization and reports of bullying behavior. Similarly, at an organizational level, particular practices of a school, such as peer coaching and peer bullying prevention skills, could be examined in terms of producing a safe school environment as identified by students, teachers, and administrators. In this respect, educational policy decisions would be based on locally valid evidence. Such an approach is especially relevant in that it targets several important barriers to the dissemination of anti-bullying interventions, including its acceptability, feasibility, and sustainability. Teacher acceptance and commitment to a program or intervention strategy, as well as the presence of a site-based facilitator to support the implementation, are among the most potent determinants of high-quality and sustained use of peer coaching and other EBP (Gersten, Chard, & Baker, 2000). Furthermore, incorporating an EBP model to examine the effects of an anti-bullying program naturally requires a data-based, problem-solving approach, which includes the effects on peers. Examining the impact of anti-bullying interventions on peers and peer group relationships is essential, as peers are viewed as holding a critical role in both the implementation and the effectiveness of bullying programs. That is, positive implementation of bullying prevention should lead to positive changes in peer behavior, including social, affective, and academic outcomes.

CONCLUSION

The real school bullying problem is complex and must incorporate an emphasis on effective intervention in schools. Such complexity requires an ecological theoretical orientation to account for it and a sustained agenda for the development of EBI strategies. In light of the significant gaps in what we know about effective bullying prevention and intervention, and the pressure for schools to intervene immediately and effectively, school psychologists and other mental health professionals working in schools must rely on innovative conceptions of effective bullying intervention in schools. Although there are potential limitations in the model proposed here, we expect that it will contribute to the conversation and work on effective interventions that address the real bullying problem in schools.

REFERENCES

Boulton, J. J., & Underwood, K. (1992). Bully/victim problems among middle school children. *British Journal of Educational Psychology, 62,* 73–87.

Bronfenbrenner, U. (1979). *The ecology of human development: Experiments by nature and design.* Cambridge, MA: Harvard University Press.

Cairns, R. B., Leung, M. C., Buchanan, L., & Cairns, B. D. (1995). Friendships and social networks in childhood and adolescence: Fluidity, reliability, and interrelations. *Child Development, 66,* 1330–1345.

Committee for Children. (2001). *Steps to respect: A bullying prevention program.* Seattle, WA: Author.

Conduct Problems Prevention Research Group. (1999). Initial impact of the fast track prevention trial for conduct problems: I. The high-risk sample. *Journal of Consulting and Clinical Psychology, 67,* 631–647.

Craig, W., & Pepler, D. J. (1997). Observations of bullying and victimization on the schoolyard. *Canadian Journal of School Psychology, 2,* 41–60.

Dishion, T. J., McCord, J., & Poulin, F. (1999). When interventions harm: Peer groups and problem behavior. *American Psychologist, 54,* 755–764.

Doll, B., Song, S. Y., & Siemers, E. (2002). Practices that neutralize bullying in elementary classrooms. In S. M. Swearer & D. Espelage (Eds.), *Bullying in the schools: A social and ecological perspective on intervention and prevention* (pp. 161–183). Mahwah, NJ: Lawrence Erlbaum.

Doll, B., Zucker, S., & Brehm, K. (2004). *Resilient classrooms: Creating healthy environments for learning.* New York: Guilford.

Farrell, A., Meyer, A., Kung, E., & Sullivan, T. (2001). Development and evaluation of school-based violence prevention programs. *Journal of Clinical Child Psychology, 30,* 207–220.

Farmer, T. W., Estell, D. B., Bishop, J. L., O'Neal, K. K., & Cairns, B. D. (2003). Rejected bullies or popular leaders? The social relations of aggressive subtypes of rural African American early adolescents. *Developmental Psychology, 39,* 992–1004.

Flannery, D. J., Wester, K. L., & Singer, M. I. (2004). Impact of exposure to violence in school on child and adolescent mental health and behavior. *Journal of Community Psychology, 32,* 559–573.

Frey, K. S., Hirschstein, M. K., Edstrom, L. V., & Snell, J. L. (2005a). *Observed reduction in bullying, victimization, and bystander encouragement: Longitudinal evaluation of a school-based intervention.* Unpublished manuscript.

Frey, K. S., Hirchstein, M. K., Snell, J. L., Edstrom, L. V. S., MacKenzie, E. P., & Broderick, C. J. (2005b). Reducing playground bullying and supporting beliefs: An experimental trial of the Steps to Respect program. *Developmental Psychology, 41,* 479–491.

Gersten, R., Chard, D., & Baker, S. (2000). Factors enhancing sustained use of research-based instructional practices. *Journal of Learning Disabilities, 33,* 445–457.

Gresham, F. M., MacMillan, D. L., Beebe-Frankenberger, M. E., & Bocian, K. M. (2000). Treatment integrity in learning disabilities intervention research: Do we really know how treatments are implemented? *Learning Disabilities Research & Practice, 15,* 198–205.

Hirschstein, M. K., Edstrom, L. V. S., Frey, K. S., Snell, J. L., & MacKenzie, E. P. (2007). Walking the talk in bullying prevention: Teacher implementation variables related to initial impact of the Steps to Respect program. *School Psychology Review, 36*, 3–21.

Hoagwood, K., & Olin, S. (2002). The NIMH blueprint for change report: Research priorities in child and adolescent mental health. *Journal of the American Academy of Child and Adolescent Psychiatry, 41*, 760–767.

Hodges, E. V. E., Boivin, M., Vitaro, F., & Bukowski, W. M. (1999). The power of friendship: Protection against an escalating cycle of peer victimization. *Developmental Psychology, 35*, 94–101.

Hodges, E. V. E., Malone, M. J., & Perry, D. G. (1997). Individual risk and social risk as interacting determinants of victimization in the peer group. *Developmental Psychology, 33*, 1032–1039.

Hodges, E. V. E., & Perry, D. G. (1999). Personal and interpersonal antecedents and consequences of victimization by peers. *Journal of Personality & Social Psychology, 76*, 677–685.

Hoover, J. H., Oliver, R., & Hazler, R. J. (1992). Bullying: Perceptions of adolescent victims in the Midwestern U.S.A. *School Psychology International, 13*, 5–16.

Kallestad, J. H. & Olweus, D. (2003). Predicting teachers' and schools' implementation of the Olweus Bullying Prevention Program: A multilevel study. *Prevention & Treatment, 6*, 1.

Kann, L., Kinchen, S. A., Williams B. I., Ross, J. G., Lowry, R., Hill, C. V., Grunbaum, J. A., Blumson, P. S., Collins, J. L., & Kolbe, L. J. (1998). *Youth risk behavior surveillance, 1997.* Atlanta, GA: Centers for Disease Control and Prevention. CDC Surveillance Summaries, August 14, 1998. MMWR; 47 (No. SS-3).

Kazdin, A. (2001). Progression of therapy research and clinical application of treatment require better understanding of the change process. *Clinical Psychology-Science and Practice, 8*, 143–151.

Kratochwill, T. R. (2006). Evidence-based interventions and practices in school psychology: The scientific basis of the profession. In R. F. Subotnik & H. J. Walberg (Eds.), *The scientific basis of educational productivity* (pp. 229–267). Greenwich, CT: Information Age.

Leff, S. S., Kupersmidt, J. B., Patterson, C. J., & Power, T. J. (1999). Factors influencing teacher identification of peer bullies and victims. *School Psychology Review, 28*, 505–517.

Limber, S., & Small, M. (2003). State laws and policies to address bullying in schools. *School Psychology Review, 32*, 445–455.

Mooney, P., Epstein, M. H., Reid, R., & Nelson, R. J. (2003). Status and trends in academic intervention research for students with emotional disturbance. *Remedial and Special Education, 24*, 273–287.

Nansel, T. R., Overpeck, M., Pilla, R. S., Ruan, W. J., Simons-Morton, B., & Scheidt, P. (2001). Bullying behaviors among U.S. youth: Prevalence and association with psychosocial adjustment. *Journal of the American Medical Association, 285*, 2094–2100.

Naylor, P., & Cowie, P. (1999). The effectiveness of peer support systems in challenging school bullying: The perspectives and experiences of teachers and pupils. *Journal of Adolescence, 22*, 467–479.

Nishina, A., Juvonen, J., & Witkow, M. R. (2005). Sticks and stones may break my bones, but names will make me feel sick: The psychosocial, somatic, and scholastic consequences of peer harassment. *Journal of Clinical Child and Adolescent Psychology, 34*(1), 37–48.

O'Connell, P., Pepler, C., & Craig, W. (1999). Peer involvement in bullying: Insights and challenges for intervention. *Journal of Adolescence, 22,* 437–452.

Olweus, D. (1991). Bully/victim problems among school children: Basic facts and effects of a school based intervention program. In I. Rubin & D. Pepler (Eds.), *The development and treatment of childhood aggression* (pp. 441–447). Hillsdale, NJ: Erlbaum.

Olweus, D., Limber, S., & Mihalic, S. F. (1999). *Bullying Prevention Program: Blueprints for Violence Prevention, Book Nine.* Blueprints for Violence Prevention Series (D.S. Elliott, Series Editor). Boulder, CO: Center for the Study and Prevention of Violence, Institute of Behavioral Science, University of Colorado.

Orpinas, P., & Horne, A. M. (2006). *Bullying prevention: Creating a positive school climate and developing social competence.* Washington DC: American Psychological Association.

Pelligrini, A. D., Bartini, M., & Brooks, F. (1999). School bullies, victims, and aggressive victims: Factors relating to group affiliation and victimization in early adolescence. *Journal of Educational Psychology, 91,* 216–224.

Pepler, D. J., Craig, W. M., Ziegler, S., & Charach, A. (1994). An evaluation of an anti-bullying intervention in Toronto Schools. *Canadian Journal of Community Mental Health, 13,* 95–110.

Pianta, R. C., & Walsh, D. J. (1996). *High-risk children in schools: Constructing sustaining relationships.* New York: Routledge.

Rodkin, P. C., & Hodges, E. V. E. (2003). Bullies and victims in the peer ecology: Four questions for psychologists and school professionals. *School Psychology Review, 32,* 384–400.

Salmivalli, C., Lagerspetz, K., Bjorkvist, K., Osterman, K., & Kaukianen, A. (1996). Bullying as a group process: Participant roles and their relations to social status within the group. *Aggressive Behavior, 22,* 1–15.

Schoenwald, S. K., & Hoagwood, K. (2001). Effectiveness, transportability, and dissemination of interventions: What matters when? *Psychiatric Services, 52,* 1190–1197.

Schwartz, D., Gorman, A. H., Nakamoto, J., & Toblin, R. L. (2005). Victimization in the peer group and children's academic functioning. *Journal of Educational Psychology, 97*(3), 425–435.

Seethaler, P. M., & Fuchs, L. S. (2005). A drop in the bucket: Randomized controlled trials testing reading and math interventions. *Learning Disabilities Research & Practice, 20,* 98–102.

Shavelson, R. J., & Towne, L. (2002). *Scientific research in education.* Washington, DC: National Academic Press.

Skiba, R., Reynolds, C., Graham, J., Sheras, P., Conoley, J. C., & Vazquez, E. (2006). *Are zero tolerance policies effective in the schools? An evidentiary review and recommendations.* A report by the Zero Tolerance Task Force. Washington DC: American Psychological Association.

Smith, D. J., Schneider, B. H., Smith, P., & Ananiadou, K. (2004). The effects of whole-school antibullying programs: A synthesis of evaluation research. *School Psychology Review, 33*, 547–560.

Snyder, P., Thompson, B., McLean, M. E., & Smith, B. J. (2002). Examination of quantitative methods used in early intervention research: Linkages with recommended practices. *Journal of Early Intervention, 25*, 137–150.

Song, S. Y. (2006). *The role of protective peers and positive peer relationships in school bullying: How can peers help?* Doctoral dissertation, University of Nebraska-Lincoln. Dissertation Abstracts International.

Song, S. Y., Doll, B., Swearer, S. M., & Johnsen, L. (2005, April). *Understanding the role of the peer ecology in bullying prevention.* Paper presented at the 2005 Annual Convention of the National Association of School Psychologists, Atlanta, GA.

Song, S. Y., Doll, B., Swearer, S. M., Johnsen, L., & Siegel, N. (in press). *How peer protection is related to school bullying: An examination of the protective peers hypothesis.* Manuscript under review.

Stephenson, P., & Smith, D. (1989). Bullying in the junior school. In D. P. Tattum & D. A. Lane (Eds.), *Bullying in schools* (pp. 45–58). Stoke on Trent: Trentham.

Stoiber, K. C., & Kratochwill, T. R. (2000). Empirically supported interventions and school psychology: Rationale and methodological issues. Part I. *School Psychology Quarterly, 15*, 75–105.

Stoiber, K. C., & Kratochwill, T. R. (2002a). Evidence-based intervention in school psychology: Conceptual foundations of the procedural and coding manual of Division 16 and the Society of the Study of School Psychology Task Force. *School Psychology Quarterly, 17*, 314–389.

Stoiber, K. C., & Kratochwill, T. R. (2002b). *Outcomes: Planning, monitoring, evaluating.* San Antonio, TX: PsychCorp.

Stoiber, K. C., & Waas, G. A. (2002). A contextual and methodological perspective on evidence-based intervention practices in school psychology in the United States. *Educational and Child Psychology, 19*(3), 7–21.

Stoiber, K. C., Lewis-Snyder, G., & Miller, M. A. (2005). Evidence-based interventions. In S. W. Lee (Ed.), *Handbook of school psychology* (pp. 196–199). Thousand Oaks, CA: Sage.

Sugai, G., & Horner, R. H. (2006). A promising approach for expanding and sustaining school-wide positive behavior support. *School Psychology Review, 35*, 245–259.

Swearer, S. M., & Doll, B. (2001). Bullying in schools: An ecological framework. *Journal of Emotional Abuse, 2*, 95–122.

Troia, G. A. (1999). Phonological awareness intervention research: A critical review of the experimental methodology. *Reading Research Quarterly, 34*, 28–51.

Twemlow, S. W., Fonagy, P., Sacco, F. C., Gies, M., Evans, R., & Ewbank, R. (2001). Creating a peaceful school learning environment: A controlled study of an elementary school intervention to reduce violence. *American Journal of Psychiatry, 158*, 808–810.

U.S. Secret Service & U.S. Department of Education. (2002). *Final report and findings of the safe school initiative: Implications for the prevention of school attacks in the United States.* Retrieved April 19, 2007, from http://www.secretservice.gov/ntac/ ssi_final_report.pdf

Weersing, V. R., & Weisz, J. R. (2002). Mechanisms of action in youth psychotherapy. *Journal of Child Psychology and Psychiatry, 43*, 3–29.

Weisz, J. R. (2000). Agenda for child and adolescent psychotherapy research: On the need to put science into practice. *Archives of General Psychiatry, 57*, 837–838.

Wolery, M., & Garfinkle, A. N. (2002). Measures in intervention research with young children. *Journal of Autism and Developmental Disorders, 32*, 463–478.

Index

Page numbers in **bold** refer to figures. Page numbers in *italics* refer to tables.